Ready Notes

to accompany

Fundamental Principles of Exercise Physiology
For Fitness, Performance, and Health

Second Edition

Robert A. Robergs, Ph.D.
University of New Mexico

Steven J. Keteyian, Ph.D.
Henry Ford Heart & Vascular Institute

Boston   Burr Ridge, IL   Dubuque, IA   Madison, WI   New York   San Francisco   St. Louis
Bangkok   Bogotá   Caracas   Kuala Lumpur   Lisbon   London   Madrid   Mexico City
Milan   Montreal   New Delhi   Santiago   Seoul   Singapore   Sydney   Taipei   Toronto

The McGraw·Hill Companies

Ready Notes to accompany
FUNDAMENTALS OF EXERCISE PHYSIOLOGY
Robert A. Robergs, Steven J. Keteyian

Published by McGraw-Hill, an imprint of The McGraw-Hill Companies, Inc., 1221 Avenue of the Americas, New York, NY 10020. Copyright © 2003 (2000) by The McGraw-Hill Companies, Inc.

2 3 4 5 6 7 8 9 0 QPD/QPD 0 9 8 7 6 5 4 3

ISBN 0-07-246218-3

www.mhhe.com

PowerPoint Presentation to accompany

Fundamental Principles Of Exercise Physiology: Fitness, Performance and Health

2nd Edition

Robert A. Robergs, Ph.D., FASEP, EPC

The University of New Mexico

&

Steven J. Keteyian, Ph.D., FACSM

Henry Ford Heart and Vascular Institute

Prepared by

Robert A. Robergs, Ph.D., FASEP, EPC

The University of New Mexico

PART 1

Energy, Metabolism, Work and Power

Chapter 1

Introduction To Exercise Physiology

What is Exercise?

A physical activity that is performed for the purpose of either improving, maintaining, or expressing a particular type(s) of physical fitness.

eg: training for or performing athletics, sports, or recreational activities such as jogging, roller blading, ice skating, swimming, etc.

What is Physical Activity?

An activity performed for purposes other than the specific development of physical fitness.

eg: activities of daily living such as shopping, gardening, house keeping, child rearing, work-related activities, etc

---

What is physical fitness?

The ability to to perform exercise and physical activity, and is usually divided into the following components:

- **cardio-respiratory endurance**

- **muscular strength**
- **body composition**

- **muscular endurance**
- **flexibility**

- **muscular power**
- **agility**

What is Exercise Training?
The repeated use of exercise to improve physical fitness.

Adaptations to Exercise
Acute adaptations
The changes in human physiology that occur during exercise or physical activity.

Chronic Adaptations
The alterations in the structure and functions of the body that occur in response to the regular completion of physical activity and exercise.

What is Exercise Physiology?

1. **An Academic Program of Study, and a Course in Exercise Science**

The study of how exercise and physical activity alter the structure and function (physiology) of the human body.

Figure 1.1

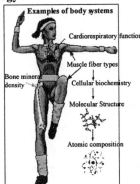

Examples of body systems

Cardiorespiratory function

Muscle fiber types

Bone mineral density

Cellular biochemistry

Molecular Structure

Atomic composition

Recent History and Development of Exercise Physiology?

1970's	2000's
PHYSICAL EDUCATION	EXERCISE PHYSIOLOGY

1970's — PHYSICAL EDUCATION
Recreation
Leisure Studies
Motor Learning
Sports Psychology
Health Education
Adapted Phys. Ed.
Biomechanics
Exercise Physiology

▼
Teacher Training

2000's — EXERCISE PHYSIOLOGY
Sports Medicine
Cardiology
Endocrinology
Pulmonology
Athletic Training
Nursing
Physical Therapy
Wellness
Occupational Therapy
Physical Education
Personal training
Physiology
Exercise Physiology

▼
Professional Employment

Table 1.1 (condensed): Applications of Exercise Physiology To Other Disciplines and Professions

Cardiology	Applications
• Biochemistry	-metabolic adaptations to muscle contraction and exercise training
• Cardiology	-diagnostics, rehabilitation, and prevention -reversal of risk factors for heart disease
• Endocrinology	-rehabilitation of type II diabetes
• Neurology	-effects of exercise on the autonomic nervous system
• Nutrition	-macro- & micro-nutrient needs during exercise, and exercise training
• Orthopedics	-effects of exercise on bone remodeling
• Physical Therapy	-injury rehabilitation/prevention
• Pulmonology	-training/conditioning of muscles used in ventilation

_____

_____

_____

_____

_____

_____

_____

Table 1.3: Examples of Prominent Researchers in Exercise Physiology (condensed)

Research Interests	Research Affiliation*
CHO and Lipid Metabolism	
David Costill	Ball State University, IN (U.S.A.)
Eddie Coyle	University of Texas-Austin (U.S.A)
Metabolic Biochemistry	
George Brooks	U.C. Berkely (U.S.A.)
Eric Hultman	Queen's Medical Center (UK)
Kent Sahlin	Karolinska Institute (Sweden)

_____

_____

_____

_____

_____

_____

Table 1.3, continued.

Research Interests	Research Affiliation*
Carbohydrate Ingestion During Exercise	
David Costill	Ball State University, IN (U.S.A.)
Eddie Coyle	University of Texas, Austin (U.S.A.)
Carl Gisolfi	deceased
Cardiovascular Function During Exercise	
Jere Mitchell	Harry S. Moss Heart Cntr. (U.S.A.)
Larry Rowell	University of Washington, Seattle (U.S.A.)
Jack Wilmore	Texas A&M University (U.S.A.)

_____

_____

_____

_____

_____

_____

_____

Table 1.3, cont.

Research Interests	Research Affiliation*
Training Adaptations	
Bengt Saltin	Karolinska Institute (Sweden)
John Holloszy	University of Washington, St Louis (USA)
Pulmonary Function/Gas Exchange/Ventilation	
Jerry Dempsey	University of Wisconsin (U.S.A.)
Eric Hultman	Queen's Medical Center (UK)
Kent Sahlin	Karolinska Institute (Sweden)

Table 1.4: Examples of journals that publish exercise physiology or related research

Journal
Acta Physiologica Scandinavia
American Journal of Physiology
Canadian Journal of Applied Sports Sciences
European Journal of Applied Physiology
International Journal of Sports Medicine
International Journal of Sports Nutrition
Journal of Applied Physiology

Table 1.4, cont.

Journal
Journal of Exercise Physiology$_{online}$
Journal of Physiology
Journal of Sports Medicine and Physical Fitness
Journal of Strength and Conditioning Research
Medicine and Science in Sports and Exercise
Professionalization of Exercise Physiology$_{online}$
Research Quarterly For Exercise and Sport
Sports Medicine

Chapter 2

**Exercise: A Challenge of
Homestatic Control**

Homeostasis: The condition of bodily function where there is a constant or unchanging internal environment.

The issues that are important in the application of homeostasis to exercise physiology are:

• how well the body can reduce the physiological consequences of the exercise stress

• the speed at which a homeostatic condition is once again attained during recovery.

A good example of the dynamic nature of homeostasis is the beat-to-beat variability in blood pressure

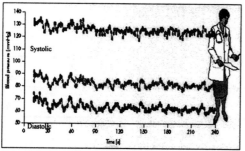

Figure 2.1

Steady state : an exercise condition where certain body functions have attained dynamic constancy at a new level. Typically, steady state is used describe the condition of a constant oxygen consumption, where the contracting muscles' energy needs are being met solely by metabolic reactions linked to the consumption of oxygen.

eg: walking, jogging, easy cycling

Figure 2.2

The changes in heart rate and oxygen consumption are good examples of physiological measures that become relatively constant during steady state exercise intensities.

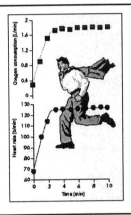

What are examples of other physiological measures that would attain a dynamic constancy during steady state exercise?

CONTROL SYSTEMS OF THE BODY

A **biological control system** is a functioning unit that works to help maintain homeostasis. The components of a biological control system are a **receptor**, **integrating control unit**, and **effector mechanism**.

In most biological control systems the response caused by the **effector mechanism** works in opposition to the initial stimulus and is termed **negative feedback**.

Gain: The precision by which a control system can prevent deviation from homeostasis.

$$Gain = \frac{Amount\ of\ correction\ needed}{Amount\ of\ abnormality\ after\ correction}$$

*A control system that has a **large gain** indicates that it has a **more sensitive regulation** that better maintains "normal" or closer to "normal" conditions.*

What are some examples of biological control systems of the human body that enable a person to perform long term (> 60 min) exercise?

Table 2.1 (condensed) : The major biological control systems of the body that are important during exercise.

Control System Effect	Stimulis/Effector	Function
↑ energy metabolism	metabolites muscle contraction	maintain cellular ATP
↑ blood glucose	↓ blood glucose	maintain blood glucose
↑ heart rate	nerves from brain, muscles, joints ↑ hormones	↑ blood flow
↑ sweat response	nerves from brain ↑ skin temp	↑ blood flow to skin ↑sweat rate ↑ heat transfer

Table 2.1, continued.

Control System Effect	Stimulis/Effector	Function
↑ lung ventilation	nerves from brain, muscles, joints ↑ blood CO2 ↓ blood O2	maintain normal blood O2 and CO2 contents; maintain blood pH
↓ peripheral vascular resistance	muscle metabolites nerves from brain ↑ muscle temp ↓ blood & tissue pH	↑ blood vessel dilation to ↓ resistance to blood flow
↑ water reabsorption in kidney	dehydration, ↑ blood osmolality, ↑ hormones	Conserve body water

Figure 2.4

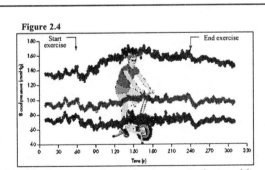

The blood pressure changes in response to the transition from rest - to steady state exercise - to a passive recovery

Feedback

Negative feedback: when the control system response works in opposition to the initial stimulus response

the majority of systems regulation in the body involves negative feedback

Positive feedback: when the control system response works to increase the initial stimulus response

Chapter 3
Metabolism

Why Study Metabolism?

The understanding of metabolism provides the directions to better understand how skeletal muscles generate energy, and how and why the body responds to exercise the way it does.

Rules of Metabolism

The study of metabolism is aided by knowing the rules of metabolism. These rules are provided by the **Laws of Bioenergetics**.

BIOENERGETICS

The study of energy transfer within the living things. There are two laws of bioenergetics.

1) *Energy cannot be created or destroyed, but can be changed from one form to another.*

2) *Energy transfer will always p roceed in the direction of increased entropy, and the release of "free energy".*

Energy that can not be reused
^ in chemical transfers reactions

ENTROPY: increased randomess or disorder.

FREE ENEGY: ΔG Energy transfer

Figure 3.1

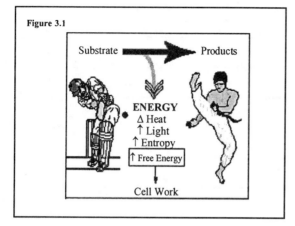

What are other examples of energy transfer within the human body or other biological systems?

Eye sight: light to electrical impulses (action potentials)

Muscle contraction: chemical energy to mechanical energy

Vitamin D formation: light energy to chemical energy

Photosynthesis: light energy to chemical energy in plants

The laws of bioenergetics can enable you to understand why these energy transfers occur.

Lessons to learn from the 1st law of bioenergetics

1. The main forms of energy within the body are;

- **heat, light, mechanical, chemical, "free energy"**, and **entropy**.

2. Entropy is a form of energy that cannot be re-used in chemical reactions, and is defined synonomously with **increased randomness** or **disorder**.

3. "Free energy" is referred to as **Gibb's free energy**, and is abbreviated "G". Typically, during energy transfers there is a change in energy forms, which is indicated by the "Δ" symbol. Thus, a change in Gibb's free energy is expressed as a "ΔG".

Lessons to learn from the 2nd law of bioenergetics

1. All reactions proceed in the direction of:
a) ↑ **entropy** ; *b)* a release of free energy (-ΔG, **(Kcal/Mol))**

2. The more negative the ΔG, the greater the release of free energy during a chemical reaction.

3. Chemical reactions that have a -ΔG are termed **exergonic reactions**.

4. By convention, reactions that require free energy input to proceed are termed *endergonic reactions*, but there are no such reactions in the human body!

- ΔG Greater the release of free energy EXERGONIC!

Requires free energy ENDERGONIC REACTION!
- but not in humans

---

5. Reactions that have not net change in substrate or product are termed **equilibrium reactions**, and have no change in free energy (ΔG=0).

6. All reactions are potentially reversible.

7. The directionality and amount of free energy release of a chemical reaction can be modified by *altering substrate and product concentrations*.
- ↑'ing products may reverse the direction of the reaction
- ↑'ing substrates can make the ΔG more negative

Of course, if the reaction is reversed, what were the products are now the substrates, and vice-versa

---

How do Cells Organize the Release and "Capture" of Free Energy During Chemical Reactions?

1. Forming ATP from reactions that release more than 14 Kcal/M of free energy (Δ G < -14 Kcal/M).

2. Using the free energy from ATP breakdown as the source of energy to make endergonic reactions exergonic .

*Most of the free energy that is released during chemical reactions **and is not used to reform ATP** is given off as heat.*

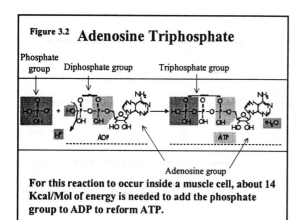

Figure 3.2 **Adenosine Triphosphate**

Phosphate group — Diphosphate group — Triphosphate group

ADP

ATP

Adenosine group

For this reaction to occur inside a muscle cell, about 14 Kcal/Mol of energy is needed to add the phosphate group to ADP to reform ATP.

Figure 3.3

Some of the **exergonic** reactions of glycolysis use ADP and ATP to "harness" free energy. ATP can then be used to provide the free energy needed to make *endergonic* reactions **exergonic**. These are examples of **COUPLING**.

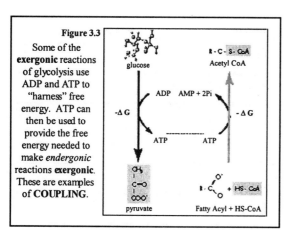

glucose

R - C - S - CoA
Acetyl CoA

ADP   AMP + 2Pi

$-\Delta G$ $-\Delta G$

ATP   ATP

pyruvate   Fatty Acyl + HS-CoA

QUESTIONS

1. Will the following reaction and direction occur by itself inside a cell?

$$ADP + Pi + H^+ \longrightarrow ATP$$

2. How much free energy is needed to make this reaction proceed in this direction inside a cell?
(what is the ΔG of this reaction?)

3. How is this "endergonic reaction" allowed to proceed inside a cell without violating the second law of bioenergetics?

Catabolism and Anabolism

Catabolism involves,

1. the breakdown of energy yielding nutrients

2. the *release of free energy and electrons* and their coupled *transfer to intermediary molecules*
    (eg. ATP, NADH + H$^+$)

3. the *formation of low energy end products*.

Overview of Catabolism   Figure 3.4, simplified

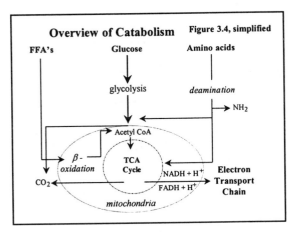

Anabolism involves the covalent bonding of electrons, protons and small molecules to produce larger molecules.

Interestingly,

- the free energy cost of building new and/or larger molecules occurs at the expense of the increased heat and entropy released from catabolism.

*- as many of the catabolic and anabolic reactions of metabolism occur together, **catabolism and anabolism function in a dynamic balance**.*

Why Are Enzymes Important?

Enzymes function as,

Biological Catalysts; the y speed up chemical reactions without being involved in the reaction or altering the free energy release.

Couplers; they provide the means to couple chemical reactions.

Regulators of Metabolism ; some can have their catalytic effectiveness either increased or decreased, thereby determining which pathway(s) is/are functional during given cellular conditions.

---

allosteric enzymes: enzymes that can be activated and inhibited.

QUESTIONS

1. What are enzymes?

2. What are the three main reasons for the importance of enzymes to cellular metabolism?

3. Are all enzymes regulated? If not, should they be?

4. Where are allosteric enzymes most likely to be located in metabolic pathways? Why?

Figure 3.5   * Allosteric enzyme

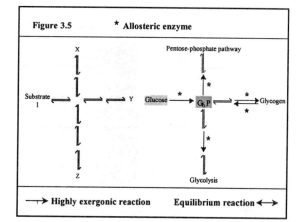

⟶ **Highly exergonic reaction   Equilibrium reaction** ⟷

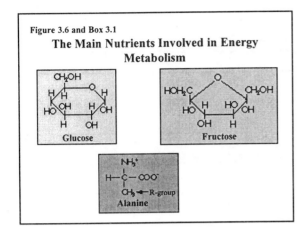

Figure 3.6 and Box 3.1

The Main Nutrients Involved in Energy Metabolism

Glucose

Fructose

Alanine

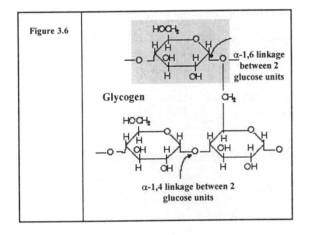

Figure 3.6

Glycogen

α-1,6 linkage between 2 glucose units

α-1,4 linkage between 2 glucose units

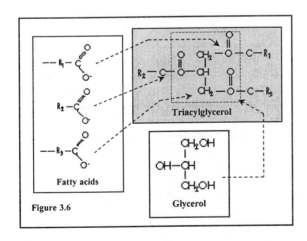

Fatty acids

Triacylglycerol

Glycerol

Figure 3.6

Figure 3.6

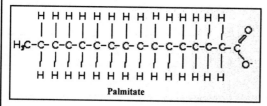

Palmitate

Palmitate is the predominant fatty acid catabolized within skeletal muscle during muscle contraction.

Figure 3.7

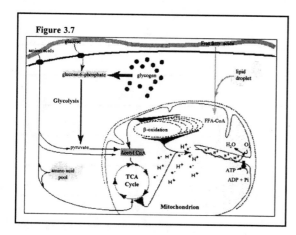

Box 3.2: Electrons, protons, and oxidation-reduction reactions.

• **Electrons** are negatively charged subatomic particles that circulate around the atom nucleus.

• Electrons are essential for atoms to form **covalent** (electron sharing) **bonds**.

• During many chemical reactions, electrons are either removed or added to molecules.

• Molecules that lose one or more electrons are *oxidized*, whereas molecules that gain electrons are *reduced*.

Consequently, *oxidation* involves the loss of electrons, and *reduction* involves the gaining of electrons.

As oxidation and reduction reactions occur together, they are often termed *oxidation-reduction* or **redox reactions**.

$$A{:}e + B \longleftrightarrow A + B{:}e$$

for example,

$$\text{pyruvate} + \text{NADH} + \text{H}^+ \xrightarrow{\textit{Lactate dehydrogenase}} \text{lactate} + \text{NAD}^+$$

Question

Which of the above molecules were reduced, and which were oxidized in the direction of lactate production?

Why are protons important?

A **proton** (H^+) is a hydrogen atom that has lost its electron.

The concentration of protons ($[\text{H}^+]$) in solution determines the acidity of the solution, and is represented numerically by the negative log of the $[\text{H}^+]$

$$(\text{pH} = -\log [\text{H}^+])$$

Thus, *a low pH represents high acidity*, and vice-versa.

Cellular pH is important to maintain (7.0 at rest), for when pH falls too far (< 6.8), electrons are forced to leave certain molecules. For proteins (eg. enzymes), this occurrence can alter the shape of the molecule, decreasing its effectiveness.

The Reactions and Metabolic Pathways of Catabolism

Skeletal muscle can produce the ATP required to support muscle contraction from one or a combination of three metabolic reactions/pathways;

1. Phosphagen System - forming ATP from using creatine phosphate or two ADP molecules

2. Glycolysis - from blood glucose or muscle glycogen

3. Mitochondrial Respiration - the use of oxygen in the mitochondria

1. The Phosphagen System

$$CrP + ADP + H^+ \xleftrightarrow{\text{creatine kinase}} ATP + Cr, \ \Delta G=0$$

The ATP production capacity of the creatine kinase reaction relies on a store of CrP, which approximates 24 mmol/kg wet wt.

$$ADP + ADP \xleftrightarrow{\text{adenylate kinase}} ATP + AMP, \ \Delta G=0$$

*Adenosine monophosphate (AMP) is the activator of the allosteric enzymes **phosphorylase** (glycogenolysis) and **phosphofructokinase** (glycolysis), thus stimulating increased carbohydrate catabolism and ATP regeneration*

Table 3.1: Examples of activities and their reliance on CrP, glycolysis, or mitochondrial respiration for ATP regeneration.

Activity	Phosph.	Glycol.	Mito.	Duration (hr:min:s)
Kicking a football	High	Low	Low	0:0:05
Pole Vault	High	Mod	Low	0:0:10
50 -100 m swim sprints	High	Mod	Low	0:0:10 - 0:0:30
400-800m run sprints	High	High	Mod	0:1:00 - 0:3:00
200 - 400m swim	High	High	Mod	0:2:00 - 0:5:00
5,000 - 10,000m run	Low	Low	High	0:12:00- 0:30:00

---

2. a) Glycogenolysis

*The catabolism of glycogen is termed **glycogenolysis**.*

$$Glycogen_n + Pi \xrightarrow{\text{phosphorylase}} Glycogen_{n-1} + Glucose\text{-}1\text{-}phosphate$$

$$Glucose\text{-}1\text{-}phosphate \xleftrightarrow{\text{phosphoglucomutase}} Glucose\text{-}6\text{-}phosphate$$

Glycogenolysis provides a rapid rate of substrate formation (G₆P) for glycolysis.

2. b) Glycolysis

During glycolysis, G_6P is produced from two sources;

1. Blood glucose

2. Muscle glycogen

Glucose entry from the blood is facilitated by specialized glucose transport proteins (*GLUT proteins*) located on and below the sarcolemma. *GLUT4 is the major transporter in skeletal muscle.*

Figure 3.10

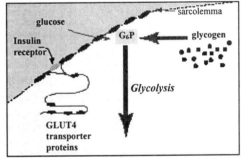

G_6P is broken down sequentially by 9 reactions that form the central carbohydrate metabolic pathway of glycolysis.

The important products of glycolysis are;

pyruvate

ATP

NADH

Pyruvate can be reduced to *lactate* in the cytosol, or be transported into the mitochondria oxidized to *acetyl Co-A*, and further catabolized by *mitochondrial respiration*.

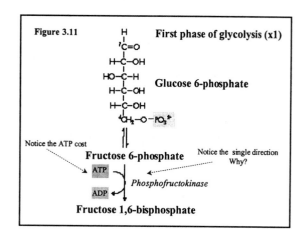

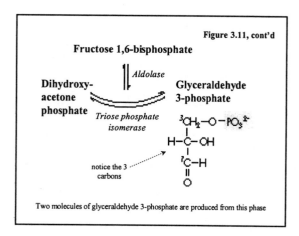

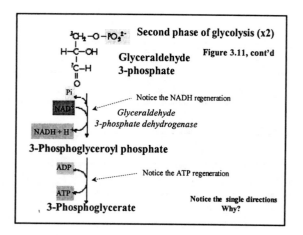

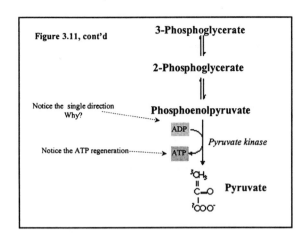

Figure 3.11, cont'd

3-Phosphoglycerate

2-Phosphoglycerate

Phosphoenolpyruvate

Notice the single direction Why?

Notice the ATP regeneration

ADP

ATP

Pyruvate kinase

Pyruvate

Lactate Production

Pyruvate can be reduced to **lactate** by the enzyme *lactate dehydrogenase* (LDH), as indicated in the equation below;

lactate dehydrogenase

$$\text{pyruvate} + \text{NADH} + \text{H}^+ \longleftrightarrow \text{lactate} + \text{NAD}^+$$
$$\Delta G = 0$$

Does lactate production also produce a proton and increase acidosis?

Is lactate production beneficial or detrimental?

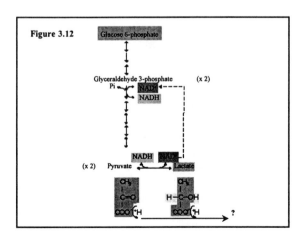

Figure 3.12

Glucose 6-phosphate

Glyceraldehyde 3-phosphate   (x 2)

Pi

NAD⁺

NADH

(x 2)   Pyruvate   NADH   NAD⁺   Lactate

?

What causes an increased production of lactate?

Lactate production will increase whenever there is a decrease in the ratio of **NAD⁺ / NADH** - termed the *redox potential*.

Conditions that will cause this are;

1. Hypoxia or ischemia (lack of oxygen delivery to the muscles).

2. When the rate of pyruvate production exceeds the rate of pyruvate entry into the mitochondria.

Understanding Acidosis

---

3. *Mitochondrial Respiration*

During pyruvate entry into the mitochondria it is converted to **acetyl CoA** by a series of linked enzymes known collectively as *pyruvate dehydrogenase*.

pyruvate dehydrogenase
Pyruvate + NAD⁺ + CoA ⟷ Acetyl CoA + NADH + H⁺ + CO₂

Acetyl Co-A can enter into a catabolic pathway called the *tricarboxylic acid cycle* (TCA cycle), which consists of 9 reactions.

The combined products of the TCA cycle are,
CO_2,
ATP,
NADH + H+,
FADH.

All of the CO_2 produced in energy metabolism can be accounted for from the pyruvate dehydrogenase reaction and 2 reactions of the TCA cycle

---

Figure 3.13

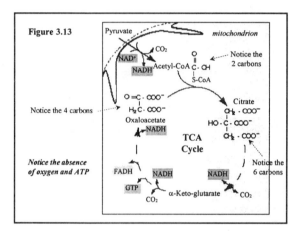

The biochemical use of oxygen, and the regeneration of ATP occurs within the mitochondria in the *electron transport chain* (ETC).

The consumption of oxygen, and formation of water and ATP during the ETC is termed *oxidative phosphorylation*.

As electrons are shuttled along the ETC, protons (H^+) are transferred into the *intermembranous space* of the mitochondria, forming a **proton gradient**. The potential "free energy" of this gradient is harnessed as protons diffuse through a special protein (**FₒF₁ protein**) within the inner membrane, providing the energy to phosphorylate ADP + Pi to ATP.

How does the NADH from glycolysis enter the mitochondria?

Cytosolic NADH does not enter the mitochondria. The electrons and protons harnessed by NADH are transferred to other molecules which can diffuse or be transported across the inner mitochondrial membrane. The "shuttling" of these electrons and protons can occur two ways:

1. glycerol-phosphate shuttle

       cytosolic NADH   mitochondrial FADH

2. malate-aspartate shuttle

       cytosolic NADH   mitochondrial NADH

Lipolysis

Lipid catabolism begins with the breakdown of triacylglycerols into fatty acids and glycerol; termed *lipolysis*.

The fatty acids that are released, or "freed" during lipolysis are referred to as *free fatty acids* (FFA). The FFAs can occur from triacylglycerols stored in *adipose tissue* or from *lipid droplets within skeletal muscle*.

FFA are catabolized within mitochondria in the pathway of β-oxidation. The products of this 4 reaction pathway are;

      acetyl CoA + NADH + FADH + FFA_{n-2} per cycle.

Does lipid burn in a carbohydrate flame within skeletal muscle?

NO. Both CHO and lipid catabolism produce acetyl CoA as the only substrate for mitochondrial respiration. Consequently, in skeletal muscle there is no means to support TCA cycle intermediates from either CHO or fat.

Amino Acid Oxidation

During catabolism amino acids can be used to form other molecules, or used to form other amino acids. For example, when the amine group is removed (deamination), it can be added to another carbon chain (transamination) to form a different amino acid.

When an amino acid is deaminated and the carbon chain is used to form a molecule of glycolysis or the TCA cycle, ATP is regenerated and the process is termed *amino acid oxidation*.

Table 3.2 simplified: Tally of ATP regeneration from catabolism.

Pathway/Reactions	ATP (net)	NADH	FADH	Total ATP
Glycolysis	2	2	0	6*
Mitochondrial Respiration (CHO)	2	8	2	30
Fatty acid oxidation (palmitate)	6	31	15	129

* assumes the glycerol-phosphate shuttle

QUESTIONS

1. Why would an increase in exercise intensity increase ATP production from CrP and glycolysis?

2. Is lactate production beneficial or detrimental to muscle function during exercise?

3. Why is the redox potential of the cytosol used to reflect the metabolic state of skeletal muscle?

4. How would an increase in mitochondrial mass in skeletal muscle influence muscle metabolism for a given exercise intensity?

5. In skeletal muscle, does lipid "burn" in a carbohydrate or amino acid "flame"?

Important Reactions and Metabolic Pathways of Anabolism

During the recovery from exercise, skeletal muscle must build molecules to restore energy reserves of glycogen and triacylglycerols, as well as repair and synthesize new proteins.

1. *Glycogen synthesis*   Notice the single ATP equivalent cost

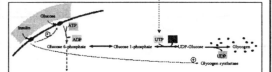

Figure 3.19

2. Triacylglycerol synthesis (in skeletal muscle)

Figure 3.20

Note that in the liver Acetyl CoA is used to synthesize fatty acids

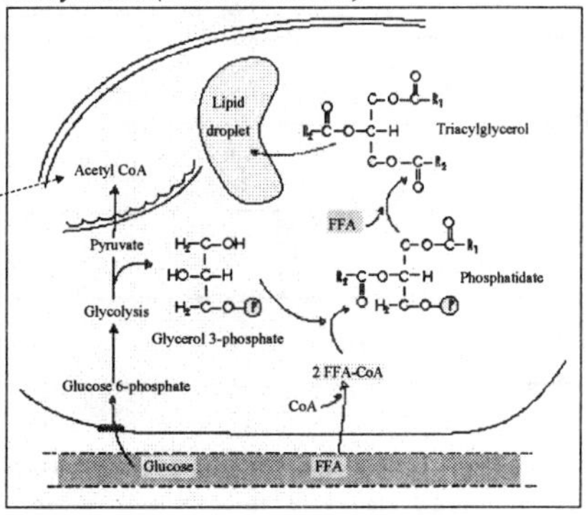

3. Amino acid and protein synthesis

Of the 20 amino acids, 10 cannot be produced in the body and must be provided by the diet: these 10 are termed *essential amino acids*.

Protein synthesis involves the processes of transcription and translation.

Transcription: the formation of ribonucleic acid (RNA) from DNA. This molecule is then processed further to form messenger RNA(mRNA).

Translation: the use of mRNA, ribosomes, and specific amino acids bound to transfer RNA (tRNA) molecules to attach amino acids to a lengthening protein chain.

Contributions of the Liver to Metabolism

The Liver

The liver is a tissue that is used to support energy provision to the tissues of the body. During exercise, the primary function of the liver is to form glucose and release it into the blood. To do this, even when liver glycogen stores become low or depleted, the liver must form glucose from non-carbohydrate molecules. The liver accomplishes this feat by the pathway of *gluconeogenesis*.

Gluconeogenesis is more than the simple reversal of glycolysis. *The live has enzymes that do not exist in skeletal muscle* so that important reactions can occur that facilitate glucose production from *lactate and certain amino acids - the main substrates for gluconeogenesis* during exercise.

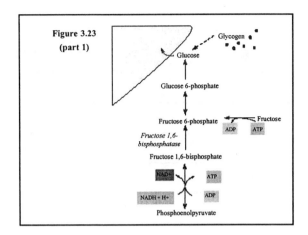

Figure 3.23
(part 1)

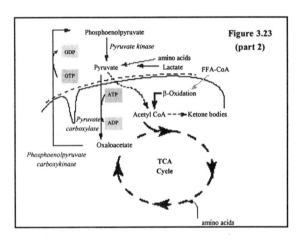

Figure 3.23
(part 2)

Chapter 4

Ergometry and Calorimetry

Ergometry

Ergometry is a science that measures work. A device that can be used to measure work is called an **ergometer**.

$$W = F \times D$$

where W = Work, F = Force, D = Distance

The **Force** must be applied against gravity, over a **Distance**

During bench stepping, body mass = *Force*, and the step height x step rate x time = *Distance*. For example;

W = 70 kg x 0.25 m/step x 30 steps/min x 30 min

= 70 kg x 225 m

= **15,750 kgm**

2

Power is work expressed relative to time. For example;

P = 15.750 kgm / 30 min

= **525 kgm/min**

You may not recognize the units of **work** and **power** used here; kgm and kgm/min, respectively.

As physical *units of work and power can be converted to other expressions of energy*, based on the first law of bioenergetics, you need to understand *how to convert the kgm unit to other units*.

3

Table C.2, Appendix C

WORK	kJ	Kcal	ft./lb	kgm
kJ	1.0	0.2388	737	1786.9
kcal	4.1868	1.0	3086	426.8
ft./lb	0.000077	0.000324	1.0	0.1383
kgm	0.009797	0.002345	7.23	1.0

The table conversion factors represent how 1 unit listed down equals the number of units listed across; eg: 1 kcal = 4.1868 kJ

[4]

Table C.2, Appendix C

POWER	kgm/min	Watts	kcal.min	kJ/min
kgm/min	1.0	0.16345	0.00234	0.00981
Watts	6.118	1.0	0.014665	0.06
kcal/min	426.78	69.697	1.0	4.186
kJ/min	101.97	16.667	0.2389	1.0

The table conversion factors represent how 1 unit listed down equals the number of units listed across; eg: 1 Watt = 6.118 kgm/min

[5]

Ergometry can be used to better understand *energy expenditure*, and the *energy cost* of performing specific exercise on ergometers.

Based on Table C.2, Appendix C;

Performing cycle ergometry at *1250 kgm/min for 45 min*;

1250 kgm/min = 204.315 Watts = 3.0 kcal/min = 12.5 kJ.min

when using kcal/min,

3.0 kcal/min x 45 min = 135 Kcals

If you think this is an unusually low energy value, you are right!!

[6]

QUESTIONS

1. Is the 135 kcals the value for biological energy expenditure, or mechanical energy production?

2. Is the body 100% efficient in converting biological energy to mechanical energy?

3. What should be larger, the biological or mechanical energy? Why?

4. What do we need to know to convert mechanical energy to biological energy expenditure?

7

The **efficiency** of the body during exercise refers to the ratio between the change in the mechanical energy produced during exercise, to the energy used to cause the exercise (biological energy expenditure).

The concept of efficiency will be defined again, and discussed in more detail, in the section on calorimetry

What Are Other Examples Of Ergometers?

Bench step (stairs) ; arm ergometer ; ? ? ? ?

Is a treadmill an ergometer ?

Does swimming involve principles of ergometry?

8

CALORIMETRY

The science that quantifies the heat release from metabolism is termed **calorimetry**.

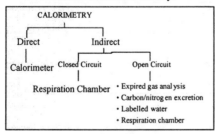

Figure 4.5

9

Definitions & Abbreviations Used in Calorimetry

VO₂ Oxygen consumption

VCO₂ Carbon dioxide production

RQ Respiratory quotient = VCO_2 / VO_2 for the cell

RER Respiratory exchange ratio = VCO_2 / VO_2 measured from expired air

Kcal/L The energy release from metabolism for each L of VO_2

Bomb Calorimeter instrument used to combust food and measure the VO_2, VCO_2, and heat release.

Respirometer instrument that quantifies the body's VO_2 and VCO_2.

10

Table 4.2: The heat release and caloric equivalents for oxygen for the main macronutrients of catabolism (*simplified*).

Food	Rubner's kcal/g	kcal/g (Bomb cal.)	kcal/g (body)	RQ	Kcal/L O₂
CHO mix	4.1	4.1	4.0	1.0	5.05
Fat mix	9.3	9.3	8.9	0.70	4.73
Protein mix	4.1	5.7	4.3	0.81	4.46
Alcohol		7.1	7.0	0.82	4.86
Mixed Diet				0.84	4.83

QUESTIONS

1. Why are the kcals/g values less for the body, especially for protein catabolism?

2. Which type of molecule provides the greatest amount of energy per mass?

3. If fat provides a greater store of energy, why does CHO provide more energy relative to VO_2?
(hint, think back to catabolism!!)

4. What is the RQ, and why is it important to assess during rest and exercise?

12

Table 4.3: The non-protein caloric equivalents for RQ (*simplified*).

RQ	Kcal/LO2	%CHO	%Fat
1.00	5.047	100	0
0.97	5.01	90.4	9.6
0.93	4.961	77.4	22.6
0.90	4.924	67.5	32.5
0.87	4.887	57.5	42.5
0.83	4.838	43.8	56.2
0.81	4.813	36.9	63.1
0.78	4.776	26.3	73.7
0.75	4.739	15.6	84.4
0.72	4.702	4.8	95.2
0.70	4.686	0.0	100

13

Open-circuit Indirect Calorimetry

When concerned with exercise, the predominant application of indirect calorimetry is for the measurement of **oxygen consumption** (VO_2). The measure is used to assess the *metabolic intensity* of the exercise.

Indirect Gas Analysis Calorimetry

Fundamental Principles

1. That the volume of oxygen consumed (VO_2) by the body is equal to the difference between the volumes of inspired and expired oxygen.

2. That the volume of carbon dioxide produced (VCO_2) by the body is equal to the difference between the volumes of expired and inspired carbon dioxide.

14

Calculating VO₂   *See Focus Box 4.1*

4.5 $$VO_2 = V_I O_2 - V_E O_2$$

as a gas volume = the volume of air multiplied by the gas fraction;

4.6 $$VO_2 = (V_I F_I O_2) - (V_E F_E O_2)$$

where $F_I O_2$ = fraction of oxygen in inspired air = 0.2093
     $F_E O_2$ = fraction of oxygen in expired air = variable

To prevent the need to measure both inspired and expired volumes, and introduce the measure of carbon dioxide, the **Haldane transformation** is used.

15

Haldane Transformation

This tranformation assumes that nitrogen is physiologically inert. Therefore, *the volume of inspired nitrogen must equal the volume of expired nitrogen*.

4.8 $\qquad (V_I F_I N_2) = (V_E F_E N_2)$

4.9 $\qquad V_I = (V_E F_E N_2) / F_I N_2$

4.10 $\qquad V_I = V_E (F_E N_2 / F_I N_2)$

where $F_I N_2$ =fraction of inspired nitrogen = 0.7903

If one neglects the rare gas component of air,

$\qquad F_E N_2 = [1-(F_E O_2 + F_E O_2)]$

Thus,

4.11 $\qquad V_I = V_E [1-(F_E O_2 + F_E O_2)] / 0.7903$

16

Incorporating equation *4.11* into *4.6* provides the final equation to calculate VO_2.

4.12 $\quad VO_2 = (V_E [1-(F_E O_2 + F_E O_2)] / 0.7903) \times F_I O_2) - (V_E F_E O_2)$

$\qquad\qquad\qquad\qquad\qquad\qquad\bullet V_I$

Calculating VCO$_2$

$\qquad\qquad VCO_2 = V_E CO_2 - V_I CO_2$

4.13 $\qquad VCO_2 = (V_E F_E CO_2) - (V_I F_I CO_2)$

where $F_I CO_2$ = fraction of carbon dioxide in inspired air = 0.0003

Calculating RER

$\qquad\qquad RER = VCO_2 / VO_2$

17

RQ vs RER

The *RQ and RER are the same measurement*, yet as the components of the measure are *obtained differently* (cell respiration vs exhaled air from the lung), under certain circumstances the *values can differ*.

The maximal range of RQ is from 0.707 to 1.0.

The range of RER may vary from <0.707 to >1.2

QUESTIONS

1. Why can RER vary so much more than RQ?

2. How do these differences alter test requirements and data interpretations?

18

The assumption of equality between RQ and RER cannot be made during the following;

1. **Metabolic acidosis** - inflates VCO_2 causing RER>1.0

2. **Non-steady state exercise** - lower than expected VO_2 and a likelihood for an inflated VCO_2 and RER.

3. **Hyperventilation** - causes a higher VCO_2 and inflates the RER.

4. **Excess post-exercise VO_2** - sustained elevated VO_2 can cause RER to be lower than expected.

5. **Prolonged exercise** - if CHO nutrition was poor and muscle and liver glycogen are low, the longer the exercise session that greater the amino acid oxidation.

19

Calculating Energy Expenditure

To calculate energy expenditure most accurately, you need to know the following;

1. **VO_2**

2. **RER**

3. **RER caloric equivalent**

4. **Exercise duration**

kcal = **VO_2** (L/min) x **RER caloric equivalent** x **time** (min)

20

For example,

when exercising at a VO_2 = 1.5 L/min and RER = 0.9 for 30 min;

kcal = **1.5** (L/min) x **4.924** x **30** (min)

= **221.6**

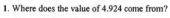

QUESTIONS

1. Where does the value of 4.924 come from?

2. Assuming all assumptions are met for calculating fat and carbohydrate contributions to energy expenditure, how much energy (kcals) came from these fuels?

3. Assuming 4 kcal/g and 9 kcal/g as the caloric densities for fat and carbohydrate, respectively, how much fat and carbohydrate were used during this exercise condition?

21

Economy vs. Efficiency

Economy - refers to the energy cost of an exercise condition.

Efficiency - the mechanical energy produced relative to the metabolic energy expenditure

For example;

The VO_2 during running is often termed "running economy" or "submaximal VO_2". A person with a lower running VO_2 for a given pace has better *economy*.

Conversely, if a person requires a smaller increase in VO_2 during a change in running pace, then that person has better *efficiency*.

Economy and efficiency can be related, but the terms should not be used interchangeably.

22

Figure 4.10

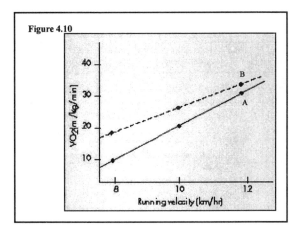

PART 2

Systemic Responses to Exercise

Chapter 5

Neuromuscular Function and Adaptations to Exercise

The Nervous System

Provides rapid communication between the brain and the different tissues and organs of the body.

Nerves - specialized cells that conduct *action potentials* along their axon.

Synapse - connection between nerves or a nerve and target tissue membrane.

Receptor - specific protein located on the membrane of a target tissue that binds to the *neurotransmitter* released by the nerve.

Functional and Anatomical Divisions of the Nervous System

Functional	Anatomical
Somatic - sensory	**Central** (CNS) - brain
- motor	- spinal cord
Autonomic - parasympathetic	**Peripheral** - nerves - efferent
- sympathetic	- afferent
	- ganglia

_____

_____

_____

_____

_____

_____

_____

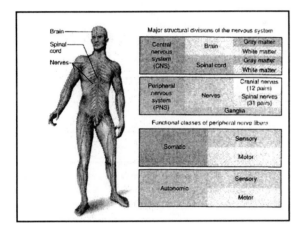

_____

_____

_____

_____

_____

_____

Table 5.1: Examples of neurotransmitters, simplified.

Neurotransmitter	Locations	Functions During Exercise
Acetylcholine	motor cortex, Aα motor nerves	↑ muscle contraction ↑ sweating
Norepinephrine	brainstem, sympathetic nerves	↑ heart rate, ↑ muscle metabolism
Epinephrine	adrenal medulla	↑ heart rate, ↑ muscle metabolism
Dopamine	basal ganglia	motor coordination
Serotonin	brainstem, spinal cord	↑ perception of fatigue
GABA	brainstem, spinal cord	motor coordination

_____

_____

_____

_____

_____

_____

_____

Nerve-Muscle Interactions

Initiating Movement

Voluntary movement requires muscle contractions that are the result of neural processes that begin within the Central Nervous System (CNS).

Motor cortex - a localized region of the outer layers of the brain responsible for the origin of neural processing of complex voluntary movement.

Cerebellum - located at the base of the posterior region of the brain, the cerebellum refines motor patterns from the motor cortex, and "stores" more simple or "well trained" motor patterns.

Corticospinal tract - region of the brain and spinal cord where the nerves conveying movement patterns are directed to the spinal cord and their respective peripheral motor nerves.

Nerve Classification

Not all nerves of the body are the same. A useful classification scheme is based on the *size (diameter) of the axon*, and the *presence of a myelin sheath* around the axon.

For example, the largest of the peripheral myelinated nerves is the motor nerve, classified as an **A** nerve. As it innervates skeletal muscle, as distinct from a variety of sensory receptors, it is also designated as an α nerve, hence the abbreviation Aα nerve.

The smallest unmyelinated (slowest conduction) nerves convey temperature sensations and are termed C nerves.

Instigating Movement

Stimulation of the Aα motor nerves results in the propagation of action potentials to skeletal muscle fibers, eventually causing muscle contraction.

The Neuromuscular Junction

The special synapse between a branch of an Aα motor nerve and the sarcolemma of a skeletal muscle fiber.

The neurotransmitter - *acetylcholine* - is released by the pre-synaptic membrane. Binding of acetylcholine to its receptor on the sarcolemma causes sodium channels to open, depolarize the sarcolemma, and continue the propagation of the action potential across and within the muscle fiber.

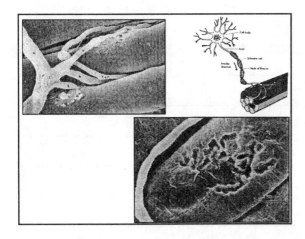

_____

_____

_____

_____

_____

_____

_____

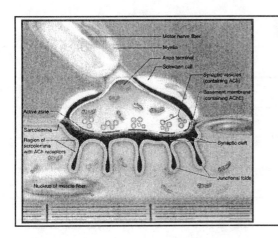

_____

_____

_____

_____

_____

_____

_____

Skeletal Muscle Contraction

Excitability - receive and propagate an action potential.

Contractility - contract/shorten

Elasticity - rapidly return to a pre-contraction length.

The demands of exercise require that skeletal muscles must be able to,

1. contract and generate a *wide range of tensions/force*,

2. alter tension/force in small increments, and

3. do this repeatedly and rapidly for durations that may vary from a few seconds to several hours.

_____

_____

_____

_____

_____

_____

_____

_____

Structure and Function Terminology

Striations -visual appearance through electron microscopy of an organized array of light and dark strands within sarcomeres.

Myofibrils -organized array of sarcomeres connected in series (end to end) along the length of a muscle fiber.

Sarcomeres -structural units of the myofiber where structural and contractile proteins are organized in a specific sequence, causing a striated appearance under electron microscopy.

Myosin - the largest of the contractile proteins

S_1 unit - the globular head region of myosin

Actin - a globular protein that forms a two stranded filament (F-actin) in vivo.

Structure and Function Terminology, cont'd.

Tropomyosin - a rod shaped protein attached to actin in a regular repeating sequence.

Troponin - a 3 component protein that is associated with each actin-tropomyosin complex.

Sarcolemma - the cell membrane of skeletal muscle.

Motor Unit - a single Aα motor nerve and all the muscle fibers that it innervates.

Table 5.2: The sequence of events during muscle contraction

When "relaxed" ADP and Pi are bound to the S_1 unit of myosin, and the unit is in the vertical "strained" position

1. depolarization of the sarcolemma and propagation of the depolarization down t-tubules to the sarcoplasmic reticulum.

2. depolarization of the triad region initiates the release of calcium into the cytosol.

3. calcium binds to troponin.

4. the troponin-calcium complex induces a conformational change in the actin-tropomyosin interaction, allowing actin to bind to myosin.

5. the actin-myosin binding allows the S_1 unit to move to the "unstrained" position, causing muscle contraction. During this process, ADP and Pi are released.

Table 5.2: The sequence of events during muscle contraction, cont'd

The binding of ATP to the S1 unit, and the immediate reaction producing ADP and Pi provides the free energy to move the S_1 unit into the "strained" position.

6. muscle contraction results from the shortening of every sarcomere in every muscle fiber of the motor units that are recruited.

7. if ATP is replenished and available, ATP binds to the S_1 unit, is broken down to ADP and Pi, and causes the S_1 unit to move to the "strained" position. ADP and Pi remain attached to the S_1 unit.

8. if calcium is still present in the cytosol due to continued neural stimulation, steps 1-7 will continue – termed *contraction cycling*.

9. Relaxation occurs when action potentials are not received at the neuromuscular junction, causing calcium to be actively pumped back into the sarcoplasmic reticulum.

Type of Contractions

Concentric

Eccentric

Isometric

Isokinetic

Figure 5.11

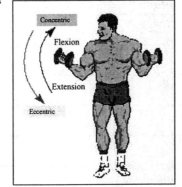

Figure 5.12

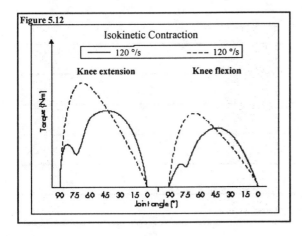

Isokinetic Contraction

—— 120 °/s   - - - - 120 °/s

Knee extension   Knee flexion

Torque [Nm]

90 75 60 45 30 15 0   90 75 60 45 30 15 0
Joint angle (°)

Length-tension Relationship

Changing muscle length, alters the degree of actin-myosin interaction, thereby influencing the tension developed during contraction.

Excessive stretch and shortening both impair tension development during contraction, producing an "inverted U" (∩) relationship between sarcomere length and contractile tension.

Force, Power and Contraction Velocity

Maximal contractile tension decreases with increases in the velocity of muscle shortening.

Maximal Voluntary Contraction (MVC) - occurs at zero velocity (isometric).

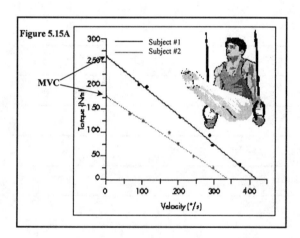

Figure 5.15A

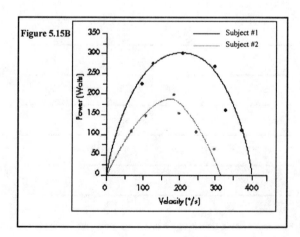

Figure 5.15B

Figure 5.15C

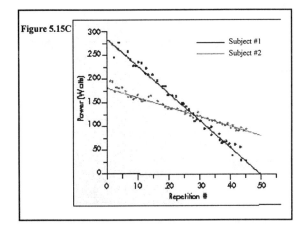

Summation - the increased contractile force resulting from the repeated stimulation of motor units at frequencies that prevent complete relaxation.

Tetanus - the continuous maximal tension resulting from when the stimulus frequency to a muscle has increased to extremely high values.

Muscle Tone - the firmness of muscle at rest due to the continual recruitment of small numbers of motor units.

Motor Units and Muscle Fiber Types

Based on research of animals (cat, dog, rat) it is known that,

1. there are *numerous differences* between the *nerves* and *muscle fiber metabolic* characteristics of skeletal muscle motor units,

2. for a given motor unit, all muscle fibers have similar metabolic profiles,

3. Both the nerve and muscle characteristics combine to differentiate motor unit types.

Table 5.3: Classification nomenclature of mammalian motor units

Classification Method	Nomenclature			
Visual	Red	White		
Contractile Velocity	Slow-twitch	Fast-twitch		
Contractile Velocity and Metabolism	I Slow-twitch	IIab Fast-twitch intermediate	IIa Fast-twitch fatigue resistant	IIb Fast-twitch fatigable
Contractile Velocity and Metabolism	S Slow-twitch	F(int) Fast-twitch intermediate	FR Fast-twitch fatigue resistant	FF Fast-twitch fatigable
Contractile Velocity and Metabolism	SO Slow-twitch oxidative		FOG Fast-twitch oxidative glycolytic	FG Fast-twitch glycolytic

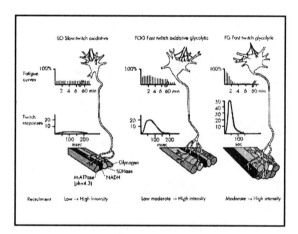

Motor Unit Recruitment

SO motor units are recruited first during exercise. As exercise intensity increases, there is a *progressive and additive* increase in *FOG and FG motor unit recruitment*. This order has been referred to as the **"size principle"**.

Electromyography

Electromyography is the study of muscle function from the detection of the electrical activity emanating from the depolarization of nerves and muscle membranes that accompany contraction.

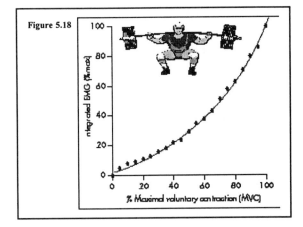

Figure 5.18

Human Muscle Biopsy and Histology

Morphological and metabolic characteristics of human muscle fibers have been researched using the method of *percutaneous needle biopsy.*

The information gained from biopsy research of human skeletal muscle includes;

1. *Muscle enzyme activities*
2. *Muscle metabolite/substrate concentrations*
3. *Muscle fiber types (myosin ATPase stain)*
4. *Muscle fiber glycogen content (PAS stain)*
5. *Muscle capillary density*
6. *Muscle damage*

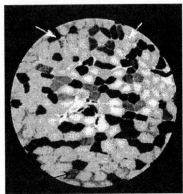

Figure 5.20A

myosin-ATPase stain

preincubation
pH=4.6

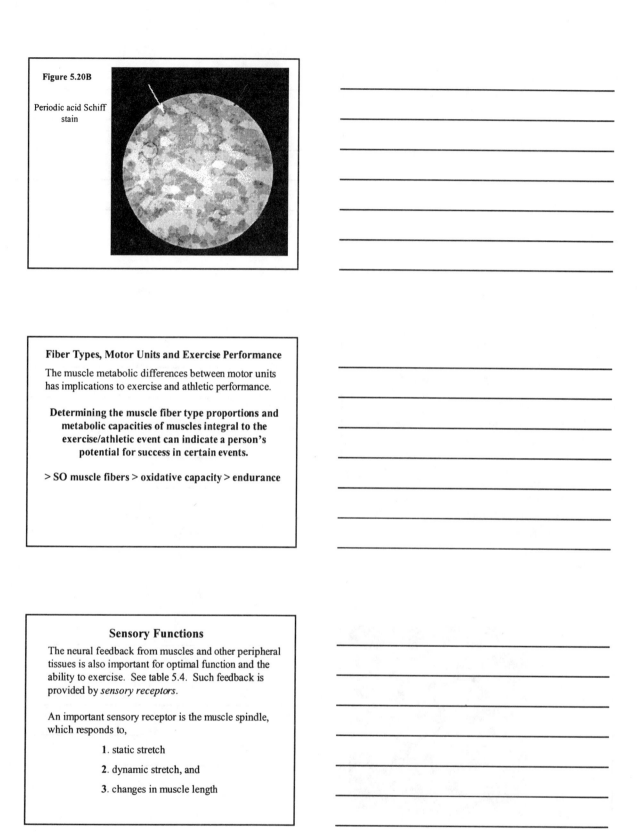

Figure 5.20B

Periodic acid Schiff stain

Fiber Types, Motor Units and Exercise Performance

The muscle metabolic differences between motor units has implications to exercise and athletic performance.

Determining the muscle fiber type proportions and metabolic capacities of muscles integral to the exercise/athletic event can indicate a person's potential for success in certain events.

> SO muscle fibers > oxidative capacity > endurance

Sensory Functions

The neural feedback from muscles and other peripheral tissues is also important for optimal function and the ability to exercise. See table 5.4. Such feedback is provided by *sensory receptors*.

An important sensory receptor is the muscle spindle, which responds to,

      1. static stretch

      2. dynamic stretch, and

      3. changes in muscle length

Table 5.4: Examples of sensory receptors of the body

Receptor	Function During Exercise
Mechanoreceptors	
Muscle Spindle	"smooth" muscle contractions, kinesthesis
Golgi tendon organ	Prevent muscle injury from excessive strain
Joint receptors	↑ Ventilation, kinesthesis
Thermoreceptors	Thermoregulation
Chemoreceptors	
Aortic and Carotid bodies	Blood O_2 and CO_2 concentrations, Regulate ventilation

---

Important Components of the Muscle Spindle

Intrafusal fibers - fibers within the muscle spindle.

Nuclear bag fiber - a type of intrafusal fiber that has nuclei located in the central enlarged region.

Nuclear chain fiber - a type of intrafusal fiber that is thinner than the bag fiber an has nuclei located along the length of the fiber.

Primary (Ia) afferent - nerve that surrounds the central region of the bag and chain fibers.

Annulospiral ending - structure formed from the wrapping of the Ia afferent nerve around an intrafusal fiber.

Gamma (γ) efferent - the type of motor nerve that innervates the contractile regions of the intrafusal fibers.

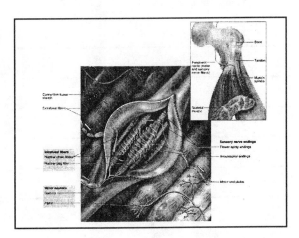

Neuromuscular Adaptations to Exercise

The dissimilar metabolic characteristics of muscle fibers from different motor units, combined with the recruitment transition from slow - to fast twitch emphasizes the need to interpret metabolic changes during exercise relative to the types of motor units recruitment.

During incremental exercise, the increasing FT motor unit recruitment results in;

- ↑ glycogenolysis

- ↑ carbohydrate oxidation

- ↑ muscle lactate production

- ↓ metabolic efficiency????

Training Adaptations

Fiber Size and Number

Hypertrophy - the increased size (x sect'l area) of skeletal muscle fibers.

Hyperplasia - the increase in the numbers of muscle fibers within a muscle.

Increases in muscle size occur mainly from hypertrophy.

Hypertrophy is greater for resistance than endurance exercise.

Hyperplasia probably occurs, but only at a small level (< 5%↑)?

Neural Adaptations

During the initial weeks of strength training, muscular strength increases without evidence of hypertrophy or hyperplasia. Why?

↑ maximal motor unit recruitment

↑ synchronous recruitment of motor units

Strength gains are also greater and more rapid when an eccentric component is used during lifting.

Atrophy

Occurs when training is stopped, and involves a decrease in muscle fiber size.

Chapter 6

Metabolic Adaptations to Exercise

Acute Adaptations

The changes in human physiology that occur during exercise, or in the recovery from exercise.

When concerned with the acute metabolic adaptations to exercise, it is important to apply an understanding of the three main sources/pathways of free energy release ;

* Creatine phosphate

* Glycolysis

* Mitochondrial respiration

Figure 6.1

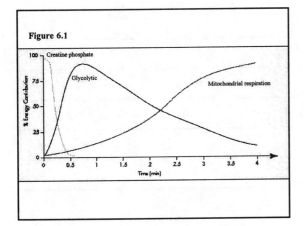

Adaptations During Incremental Exercise

An important type of exercise in exercise physiology is **incremental exercise** - involves repeated increments in exercise intensity over time.

Incremental exercise protocols can vary in the duration at each specific intensity (stage), and the magnitude of each increment.

The specific nature of the acute metabolic adaptations to incremental exercise depend on the;

type of exercise,

the magnitude of the increase in intensity/stage, and

the duration of each stage

Maximal Oxygen Consumption (VO_2max)

The maximal rate at which the body can consume oxygen during exercise.

The measurement of VO_2max is a fundamental concept in exercise physiology, and must be understood as a prerequisite for further study of metabolic and systemic physiological changes during exercise.

VO_2max is typically measured near/at the end of an incremental exercise protocol to volitional fatigue.

Criteria used to ascertain the attainment of VO_2max include;

- Plateau in VO_2
- RER > 1.1
- HR within 10 b/min of estimated (220-age)

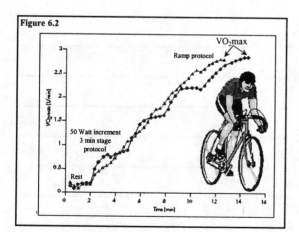

Figure 6.2

Units of VO$_2$max

VO$_2$max can be expressed as either;

☞ L/min

☞ mL/kg/min

☞ mL/kg LBM/min

☞ mL/kg$^{0.75}$/min

The unit used depends on either,

the mode of exercise,

the subject characteristics (gender, age)

the purpose of any comparison in VO$_2$max values

(male vs female)

What Determines VO$_2$max?

Many physiological and metabolic capacities contribute to VO$_2$max. It is generally accepted that a person's *VO$_2$max is indicative of their maximal cardiorespiratory capacities.* However, other variables will influence VO$_2$max, and these include;

❧ health/disease

❧ genetics (motor unit proportions, heart size, hematology)

❧ training status

❧ exercise mode

❧ muscle mass exercised

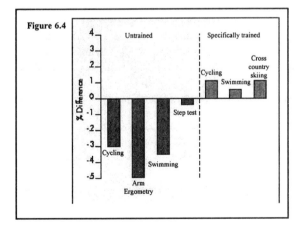

Figure 6.4

Figure 6.5

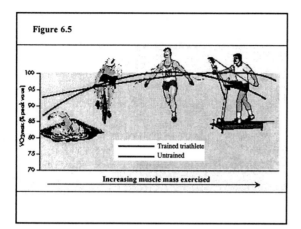

Controversy over the measurement of VO_2max

Some physiologists believe that *VO_2max may not be a true maximal value*, but a peak value that occurs due to the fatigue associated with incremental exercise to volitional fatigue.

The rationale used to justify this belief includes;

1. Not all individuals attain a plateau in VO_2 at VO_2max

2. Research is not clear in identifying limitations in oxygen delivery at VO_2max.

However, it is generally accepted that a VO_2max does exist, but may not be attained in certain individuals.

The individuals who are more likely to attain a VO_2peak rather than VO_2max are;

   ↖ Prepubescent children

   ↖ Sedentary individuals

   ↖ Individuals with acute illness (cold, flu, asthma)

   ↖ Individuals with disease (CHD, diabetes)

% VO2max: A Relative Measure of Exercise Intensity

Exercise intensities can be expressed as a percent (%) of VO_2max, and then compared between individuals or before and after an intervention (eg. training).

Metabolic Adaptations to Incremental Exercise

As exercise intensity increases there is an,

↑ catabolism of creatine phosphate

↑ catabolism of carbohydrate
(blood glucose and muscle glycogen)

↓ catabolism of lipid

↓ muscle redox potential (NAD⁺ / NADH)

↑ acidosis

↑ production of lactate

Many of these changes exhibit a threshold pattern

Lactate Threshold

Refers to the exercise intensity where there is an abrupt increase in either of muscle or blood lactate.

Figure 6.8B

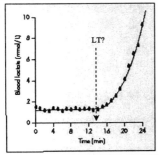

To improve the detection of this threshold, researchers transform the lactate values to their log_{10} expression.

Figure 6.8A

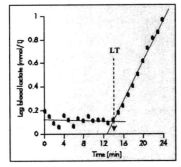

What causes the LT?

- ❖ ↑ Production of lactate
- ❖ ↑ Removal of lactate
- ❖ ↑ Fast twitch motor unit recruitment
- ❖ Imbalance between glycolysis and mitochondrial respiration
- ❖ Ischemia
- ❖ Muscle hypoxia
- ❖ ↓ Redox potential (NAD^+ / NADH)

Other Lactate Threshold Terminology

Anaerobic threshold - first used in 1964 and based on increased blood lactate being associated with hypoxia. Now known to be an oversimplification, and should not be used.

Onset of blood lactate accumulation (OBLA) - the maximal steady state blood lactate concentration, which can vary between 3 to 7 mmol/L.

Research has shown that there is considerable similarity in each of the exercise intensities obtained from the different lactate threshold methodologies.

Remember that the limitation to exercise above the LT is not the increased blood and muscle lactate but the associated increase in acidosis and other markers of muscle fatigue.

QUESTIONS

1. What do researchers currently do to verify that a VO_2max was attained?

2. Why are there so many units to express VO_2max?

3. What are the variables that will influence VO_2max?

4. Why do exercise physiologists measure VO_2max?

5. Why do exercise physiologists measure the LT?

Adaptations During Steady State Exercise

a. Oxygen Kinetics

Note the slower response time to steady state for untrained

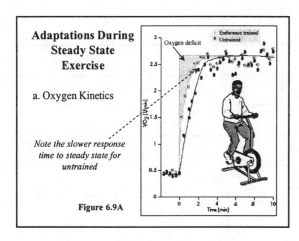

Figure 6.9A

Note the faster response time but slightly delayed steady state for larger intensity increments

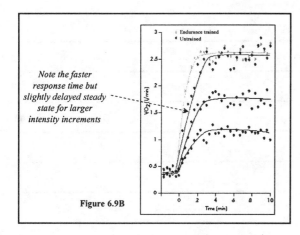

Figure 6.9B

b. VO$_2$ Drift

For exercise intensities > 60% VO$_2$max, prolonged exercise (> 30 min) causes a slight continued increase in VO$_2$.

c. CHO Catabolism

Increases with an increase is exercise intensity, with an increasing reliance on muscle glycogen.

d. Lipid Catabolism

Decreases with an increase is exercise intensity. The majority of the source of FFA used during exercise is from intramuscular lipid droplets.

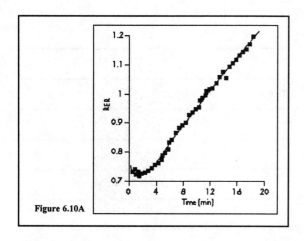

Figure 6.10A

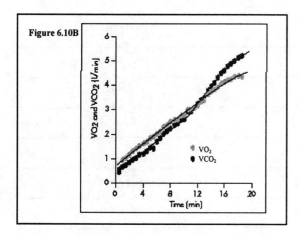

Figure 6.10B

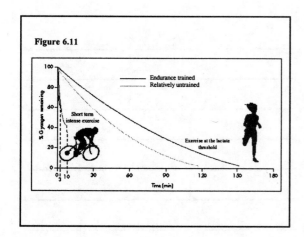

Figure 6.11

8

e. Amino acid and ketone body catabolism

Amino acid catabolism an contribute up to 10% of energy expenditure with

- ↑ exercise intensity
- low muscle glycogen and blood glucose
- ↑ duration of exercise

Amino acid catabolism serves to,

1. Provide carbon skeletons for catabolism *(also ketone bodies)*

2. Supplement TCA cycle intermediates

3. Provide gluconeogenic precursors for the liver
(also ketone bodies)

Figure 6.12 a, b

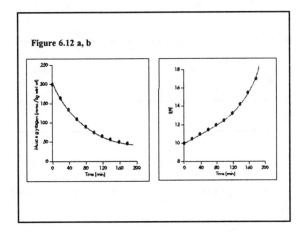

Figure 6.12 a, c

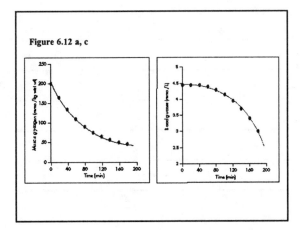

Metabolic Adaptations to Intense Exercise

During intense exercise,

☞ VO$_2$ ↑ rapidly (Fig 6.13)

☞ CrP ↓ rapidly (Fig 6.14)

☞ low muscle glycogen does not seem to impair intense exercise

☞ there is an ↑ in alanine production and release

☞ there is an ↑ in ammonia production and release

☞ there is an ↑ in lactate production and release

☞ there is an ↑ in muscle and blood acidosis

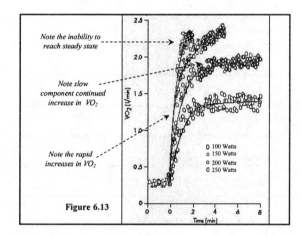

Note the inability to reach steady state

Note slow component continued increase in VO$_2$

Note the rapid increases in VO$_2$

□ 100 Watts
○ 150 Watts
○ 200 Watts
◐ 250 Watts

Figure 6.13

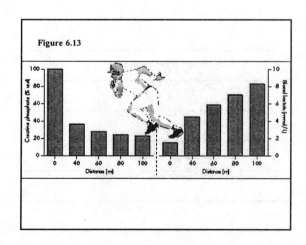

Figure 6.13

Anaerobic Capacity

The capacity of a person's ability to regenerate ATP from CrP, ADP and glycolysis.

Although difficult to measure, an accepted method for estimating the anaerobic capacity is the **accumulated O₂ deficit** (AOD).

The AOD is larger in sprint trained athletes than endurance trained athletes

Figure 6.15

Notice the rapid and sustained dependence on glycolysis

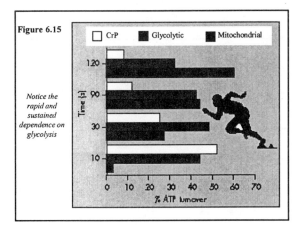

Recovery From Steady State Exercise

As most activities are not continuous, understanding the recovery from exercise has important applications sports, athletics and daily living.

a. *Excess Post-exercise VO₂* (**EPOC**)
After exercise is stopped, there is a sustained elevated VO₂ (EPOC). EPOC is caused by

- ❖ CrP regeneration
- ❖ lactate oxidation
- ❖ glycogen synthesis
- ❖ protein synthesis
- ❖ blood reoxygenation
- ❖ ↑ body temperature
- ❖ ↑ heart rate
- ❖ ↑ ventilation
- ❖ ↑ circulating hormones

Figure 6.16

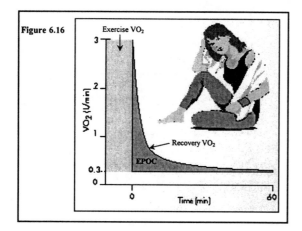

---

b. *Glycogen Synthesis*

&ζ Greater synthesis occurs during a passive recovery

&ζ Maximal synthesis requires CHO ingestion (0.7 g/kg/Hr)

&ζ Muscle damage caused by exercise slows glycogen synthesis

&ζ An active recovery prevents synthesis in slow twitch fibers.

c. *Triacylglycerol Synthesis*

Little is known of post-exercise muscle triacylglycerol synthesis. However, it is assumed that muscle triacylglycerols are restored in the recovery.

Recovery From Intense Exercise

At the end of intense exercise, muscle metabolism differs to steady state conditions;

- near maximal blood flow
- larger increases glycolytic intermediates
- larger increase in muscle lactate
- larger increases in muscle temperature
- larger increases in catecholamine hormones

These different muscle metabolic conditions result in,
- \> EPOC
- \> rate of glycogen synthesis
- prolonged time to maximal blood lactate concentrations
- delayed recovery of CrP with increased acidosis

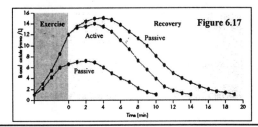

Figure 6.17

Figure 6.18 a,b

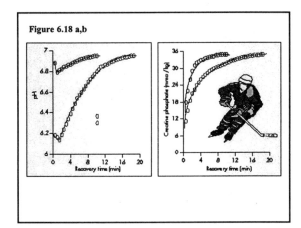

QUESTIONS

1. Why is recovery from intense exercise important for improved sports performance?

2. What would be a better recovery from intense exercise - active or passive? Why?

3. What are examples of sports or athletic events where individuals do not use appropriate recover conditions between bouts?

Chronic (Training) Adaptations

Table 6.1: Muscle metabolic adaptations resulting from training for long term muscular endurance

Metabolic Pathway	Adaptation	Consequence
Mitochondrial respiration	↑ Number & size of mitochondria	↑ Rate of mitochondrial respiration ↑ Capacity to oxidize CHO ↑ Sensitivity to stimulation ↓ Oxygen deficit ↓ Lactate production
	↑ Activity of TCA cycle enzymes	↑ Capacity to oxidize acetyl CoA

Table 6.1:, cont'd.

Metabolic pathway	Adaptation	Consequence
Mitochondrial respiration	↑ Activity of β–oxidation enzymes	↑ Capacity to oxidize lipid sparing of muscle glycogen
Glycogen	↑ Concentration	↑ time to exhaustion
Glycolysis	↑ Activity of phosphorylase ↑ LT	↑ Capacity of glycolysis ↑ Maximal steady state
	↑ Lactate removal	↑ Capacity to normalize blood & muscle lactate
	↓ Lactate production	↓ Acidosis

Table 6.1:, cont'd.

Metabolic pathway	Adaptation	Consequence
Creatine phosphate	↑ Threshold	↑ Maximal steady state
Buffering capacity	No change	

14

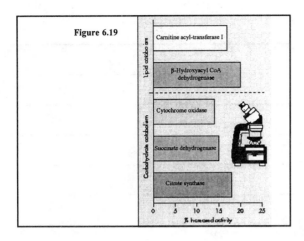

Figure 6.19

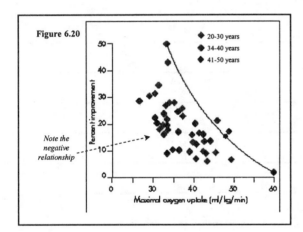

Figure 6.20

Note the negative relationship

Additional Adaptations

Metabolic thresholds - increase independent of VO_2max.

Running economy - can improve ($\downarrow VO_2$) with long term training.

Muscle glycogen stores - increase

QUESTIONS

1. Why is the increase in mitochondrial mass so important?

2. Which of the chronic adaptations are more important for improving performance? Why?

Table 6.2: Muscle metabolic adaptations resulting from training for short term muscular strength and power

Metabolic pathway	Adaptation	Consequence
Mitochondrial respiration	Small ↑	May improve recovery
Glycogen	↑ Concentration	↑ Fuel for glycolysis
Glycolysis	↑ Activity of phosphorylase	↑ Rate of glycolysis
	↑ Activity of PFK	↑ Rate of glycolysis
ATP	Small ↑	↑ Tolerance of intense exercise

Table 6.2:, cont'd.

Metabolic pathway	Adaptation	Consequence
Creatine phosphate	Small ↑	↑ Capacity to rapidly regenerate ATP
Buffering capacity	↑ Capacity	Delays fatigue from acidosis ↑ ATP from glycolysis

Figure 6.21

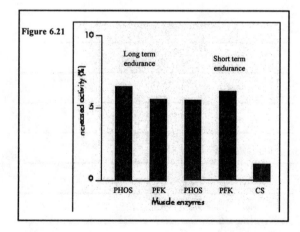

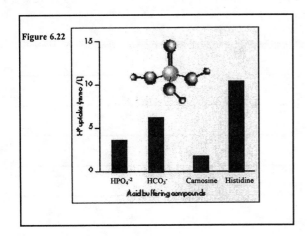

Figure 6.22

Chapter 7

Cardiovascular Function and Adaptation to Exercise

Components of the Cardiovascular System

The cardiovascular system is composed of *blood*, the *heart*, and the *vasculature* within which blood is pumped throughout the body.

Pulmonary circulation - concerning blood flow to, within and from the lungs

Systemic circulation - concerning blood flow to, within and from the remainder of the body, and consists of tissue/organ specific circulation beds, eg: *renal, hepatic, cranial, gastric, intestinal, skeletal muscle, cutaineous*, etc.

Blood

Cell component - red and white blood cells, and platelets constitutes ~45% of blood volume = hematocrit

polycythemia - excess production of red blood cells causing an abnormal increase in red blood cells

anemia - abnormally low red blood cell counts

Liquid component - water, clotting proteins, transport proteins, lipoproteins, glucose, fatty acids, antibodies, transferrin, waste products (eg. urea, ammonia, etc.), etc.

plasma - the liquid component of blood and all of it's non-cellular content

serum - what remains of plasma after blood has clotted.

Blood volume approximates 5 L, but varies in proportion to body size, endurance training status, and exposure to extreme environments (hypobaria, hyperbaria, heat, etc.)

5 L = plasma volume (PV) + cell volume (hematocrit)
   = (0.55 x 5) + (0.45 x 5)
    = 2.75 + 2.25

For young men aged 18-35, PV can be estimated from,

$$PV \text{ (L)} = 0.042 \times LBM \text{ (kg)} + 0.567 \qquad \textbf{(7.1)}$$

The molecules dissolved in plasma determine plasma **osmolality**, which is similar for all body fluids at 285-295 mOsmol/kg

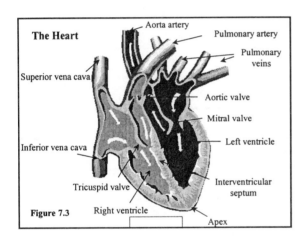

The Heart

Figure 7.3

Aorta artery
Pulmonary artery
Pulmonary veins
Superior vena cava
Aortic valve
Mitral valve
Left ventricle
Inferior vena cava
Interventricular septum
Tricuspid valve
Right ventricle
Apex

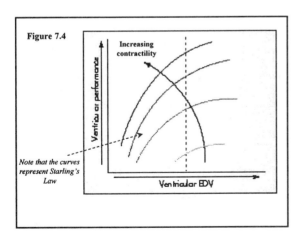

Figure 7.4

Increasing contractility

Ventricular performance

Note that the curves represent Starling's Law

Ventricular EDV

Important terminology

Cardiac cycle - the cycle of blood flow and related electrical and mechanical events as blood is received and ejected by the heart.

Preload - the stretch on the ventricular myocardium at end-diastolic volume.

Afterload - the pressure that must be overcome by the ventricles prior to ejection (= DBP for the left ventricle).

Frank-Starling Law - concerns the increase in the velocity/power of myocardial contraction with increasing stretch/EDV.

Contractility - concerns the increase in the velocity/power of myocardial contraction at a given EDV with increasing sympathetic/catecholamine stimulation.

Stroke volume - the volume of blood ejected from the ventricles/beat.

Ejection fraction - the fraction of EDV that is the stroke volume.

Cardiac output (Q) - the volume of blood pumped by the heart each minute

$$Q \text{ (L/min)} = SV \text{ (L)} \times HR \text{ (b/min)}$$

for example,   5 L/min = 0.01 x 50 b/min   (rest conditions)

Fick equation - equation based on VO_2, Q and the arterial-venous O_2 difference

for example, $VO_2 = Q \times a\text{-}vO_2\Delta$

0.25 L/min = 5 L/min x 0.05 L   (rest conditions)

QUESTIONS

1. Why is blood is an important component of the cardiovascular system?

2. What determines blood osmolality?

3. In what ways does myocardium differ from skeletal muscle?

4. Why does the muscle mass of the left and right ventricle differ?

5. Why is an increase in contactility so important to heart function during exercise?

Acute Adaptations to Exercise

With the start of exercise, cardiovascular function changes by,

◆ ↑ heart rate
◆ ↑ ejection fraction
◆ ↑ stroke volume
◆ ↑ cardiac output
◆ redistribution of Q in favor of contracting skeletal muscle
◆ ↓ vascular resistance
◆ ↑ muscle blood flow

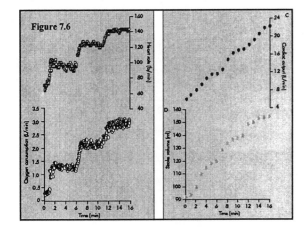

Figure 7.6

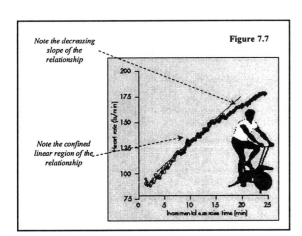

Figure 7.7

Note the decreasing slope of the relationship

Note the confined linear region of the relationship

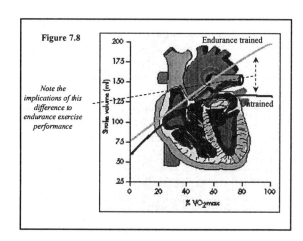

Figure 7.8

Note the implications of this difference to endurance exercise performance

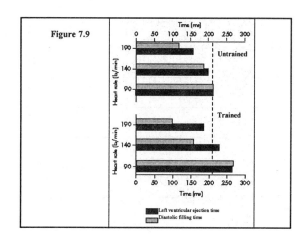

Figure 7.9

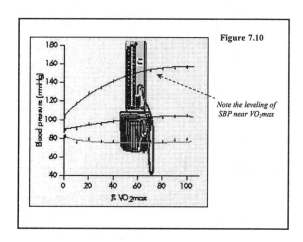

Figure 7.10

Note the leveling of SBP near VO₂max

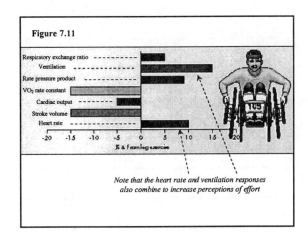

Figure 7.11

Note that the heart rate and ventilation responses
also combine to increase perceptions of effort

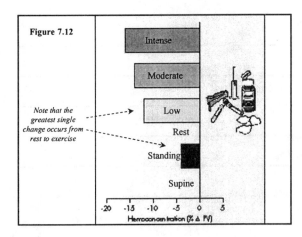

Figure 7.12

Note that the
greatest single
change occurs from
rest to exercise

Blood Flow Redistribution

Due to limitations in maximal cardiac output and blood
volume, vascular regulation enables a preferential increase
in the proportion of the cardiac output that perfuses working
skeletal muscle.

For example, muscle receives *5% of Q at rest*, but can
receive *85% of Q during intense exercise.*

Hyperemia - ↑ blood flow

Vasodilation - ↑ diameter of a blood vessel.

Vasoconstriction - ↓ diameter of a blood vessel.

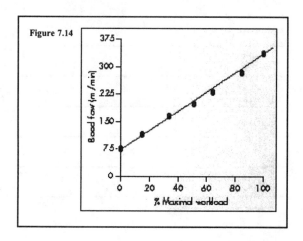

Figure 7.14

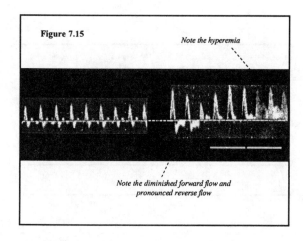

Figure 7.15

Note the hyperemia

Note the diminished forward flow and pronounced reverse flow

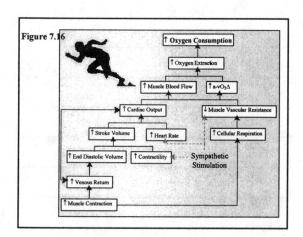

Figure 7.16

Chronic Adaptations to Exercise

Cardiovascular adaptations to training are extremely important for improving endurance exercise performance, and preventing cardiovascular diseases.

The more important of these adaptations are,

⊙ ↑ plasma volume

⊙ ↑ red cell mass

⊙ ↑ total blood volume

⊙ ↓ systolic and diastolic blood pressures

⊙ ↑ end diastolic dimensions and ventricular volumes

⊙ ↑ maximal stroke volume

⊙ ↑ maximal cardiac output

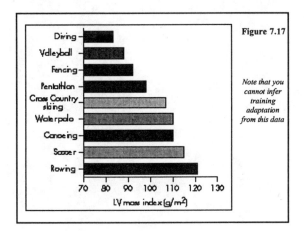

Figure 7.17

Note that you cannot infer training adaptation from this data

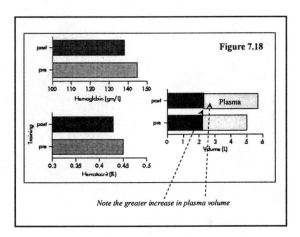

Figure 7.18

Note the greater increase in plasma volume

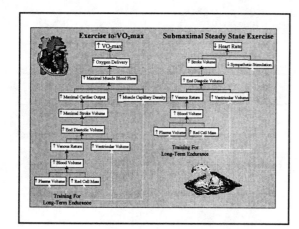

Chapter 8

Pulmonary Adaptations to Exercise

The Respiratory System

Conducting zone - consists of the mouth, nasal cavity and passages, pharynx and trachea which collectively *connect the respiratory zone of the lung to the atmospheric air* surrounding the body.

Respiratory zone - consists of the respiratory bronchioles, aveoli ducts, and alveoli which collectively represent the *sites of pulmonary gas exchange.*

Pulmonary circulation - artery, arteriole, capillary and vein network that directs blood flow from the right ventricle of the heart to the lungs, and back to the left atrium of the heart.

Note;

The conducting zone is the region of greatest resistance.

The respiratory zone has the greatest surface area and a dense capillary network.

Distribution of surfactant is aided by holes that connect alveoli called pores of Kohn.

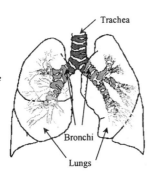

Trachea

Bronchi

Lungs

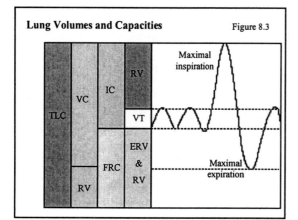

Lung Volumes and Capacities   Figure 8.3

Ventilation

The movement of air into and from the lung by the process of bulk flow.

Ventilation (V_E) (L/min) = frequency (br/min) x tidal volume (L)   **(8.1)**

For rest conditions,

V_E (L/min) = 12 (br/min) x 0.5 (L) = 6 L/min

For exercise at VO_2max,

V_E (L/min) = 60 (br/min) x 3.0 (L) = 180 L/min

Compliance - *the property of being able to increase size or volume with only small changes in pressure.*

Alveolar Ventilation

The volume of "fresh" air that reaches the respiratory zone of the lung.

Alveolar Ventilation (V_A) (L/min)

V_A = frequency (br/min) x (tidal volume - 0.15) (L)

For normal breathing conditions,

V_A = 12 (br/min) x (1.0 - 0.15) (L)   **(8.2a)**

= 12 x 0.85 = 10.2 L/min

For rapid shallow breathing conditions,

V_A = 60 (br/min) x (0.2 - 0.15) (L)   **(8.2b)**

= 60 x 0.05 = 3.0 L/min

Surfactant

A phospholipoprotein molecule, secreted by specialized cells of the lung, that *lines the surface of alveoli and respiratory bronchioles.* Surfactant *lowers the surface tension* of the alveoli membranes, *preventing the collapse* of alveoli during exhalation and *increasing compliance* during inspiration.

Respiration

The process of gas exchange, which for the human body involves oxygen (O_2) and carbon dioxide (CO_2).

> **Internal respiration** - at the cellular level

> **External respiration** - at the lung

Gas Partial Pressures in Atmospheric and Alveolar Air

Gas	Air* Fraction	Air* Partial Pressure	Alveolar Fraction^	Alveolar Partial Pressure
H_2O	0	0	----	47
O_2	0.2093	159.0	0.1459	104
CO_2	0.0003	0.3	0.0561	40
N_2	0.7903	600.6	0.7980	569

* assumes dry air
^ note that the water vapor pressure is removed to calculate alveolar gas fractions

---

Diffusion of Gases

The gases of respiration (O_2 and CO_2) diffuse down pressure gradients that exist between,

a. pulmonary blood and the alveoli

b. systemic capillary blood and cells

The factors that govern the directionality and magnitude of gas diffusion are,

■ the gas diffusion capacity

■ the gas partial pressure gradient

■ characteristics of the medium through which diffusion occurs (hydration, thickness, cross sectional area)

Transport of Oxygen in the Blood

Oxygen is transported in blood bound to **hemoglobin** (Hb). 1 gram of Hb can maximally bind 1.34 mL of oxygen (1.34 mL O_2/g Hb @ 100% saturation).

Table 8.1: Examples of hemoglobin (Hb) and oxygen carrying capacity conditions (98% saturation and pH = 7.4)

Population/Condition	[Hb]	mL O_2/L
Males	14.0	183.8
Females	12.0	157.6
Blood Doping	18.0	236.4
Anemia	< 10.0	< 131.3

[Hb] = g/100 mL

The oxygen content (CaO_2) of blood can be calculated by;

CaO_2 = [Hb] x O_2/g Hb x Hb-O_2 saturation   (8.3)

= 150 g/L x 1.34 mL O_2/g x 0.98

= 197 mL O_2/L

Another small source of oxygen in blood is the volume of *oxygen dissolved in plasma*. However, due to the low solubility of oxygen, this value is small and approximates,

dissolved O_2 = 0.003 mL / 100 mL blood / mmHg PO_2

~ 0.3 mL / 100 mL at sea level (PaO₂ ~ 100 mmHg)

Figure 8.6   *Note the relatively flat region of the curve*

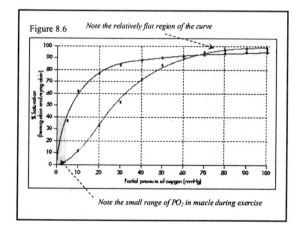

Note the small range of PO_2 in muscle during exercise

Transport of Carbon Dioxide in the Blood

The volume of CO_2 in the blood is approximately 10-fold greater than O_2.

Transport Location	Form	Percentage
Plasma	Dissolved	5
(<10%)	$CO_2 + H_2O \rightarrow H_2CO_3 \rightarrow H^+ + HCO_3^-$	<1
	Bound to proteins	5
Red Blood Cell	$CO_2 + H_2O \rightarrow H_2CO_3 \rightarrow H^+ + HCO_3^-$	65
(90%)	Dissolved	5
	Bound to hemoglobin	20

Acidosis

Quantified by the pH scale, where pH equals the negative logarithm of the hydrogen ion concentration ($[H^+]$)

$$pH = -\log [H^+] \quad \text{or} \quad [H^+] = 10^{-pH}$$

Normal blood pH is ~7.4.
The main determinants of blood pH are;
* Rate of acid production
* Concentration of HCO_3^- and other bases or acids
* $PaCO_2$
* Ventilation
* Renal excretion of acids and bases

Acute Adaptations of Pulmonary Function During Exercise

After the onset of exercise there is;
◀ a rapid ↑ in ventilation

◀ a similar rapid ↑ in pulmonary blood flow

◀ an improved V_E vs Q relationship in the lung

◀ ↑ lung compliance

◀ airway dilation and ↓ resistance to air flow

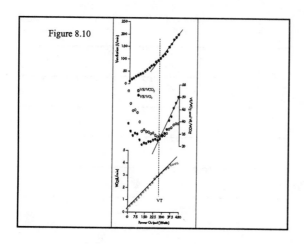

Figure 8.10

_____
_____
_____
_____
_____
_____

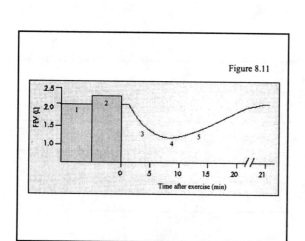

Figure 8.11

_____
_____
_____
_____
_____
_____

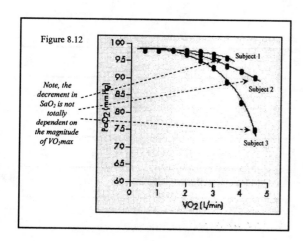

Figure 8.12

Note, the decrement in SaO2 is not totally dependent on the magnitude of VO2max

_____
_____
_____
_____
_____
_____

6

Chapter 9

Endocrine Adaptations to Exercise

Neuroendocrinology is the study of the combined function of the nerves and glands that release *hormones into the body.*

A gland is a tissue that secretes a substance within or from the body:

Exocrine glands - secrete substances from the body via a duct (eg. sweat gland, sebaceous gland)

Endocrine glands - are ductless and secrete hormones directly into the blood (eg. pancreas, adrenal, pituitary). However, *there are many examples of hormones that are not secreted from true endocrine glands* (Table 9.1).

Hormone Classification

Amine Hormones - derived from a single amino acid

Peptide Hormones - derived from amino acid peptides

Amine and peptide hormones are *water soluble*, have a *short half-life*, and exert their action via binding to a *membrane-bound receptor*. The receptor mediated response *alters cell enzyme activity* and causes a relatively *quick response time*.

Steroid Hormones - derived from the chemical structure *steroid nucleus*. Steroid hormones are transported in the blood *bound to a protein molecule*, have a relatively *long half life*, and exert their function by altering nuclear function causing a *relatively long response time*.

Table 9.1: Traditional glands and hormones, simplified

Tissue/Gland	Amine	Peptide	Steroid
		HORMONES	
Traditional			
Pituitary Anterior		LH, FSH, PRL, GH, ACTH, β-END, TSH	
Pituitary Posterior		ADH, OXYT	
Adrenal Cortex			CORT, ALD, ANDROST
Adrenal Medula	EPI, NEPI		
Testes			TEST, ESTR, ANDROST
Ovaries			ESTR, TEST, ANDROST, FSH-RP

Table 9.1: Non-traditional glands and hormones, simplified

Tissue/Gland	Amine	Peptide	Steroid
		HORMONES	
Non-traditional			
Hypothalamus		ACTH-RH, TRH, LHRH, GHRH	
Heart		ANP	
Kidney		EPO, RENIN	
Liver		IGF-1	
Lymphocytes		Interleukins	
Vascular endothelium		ET, NO (EDRF)	

Acute adaptations of the Neuroendocrine System to Exercise

The body's neuroendocrine responses to exercise are varied, multifaceted, and therefore very complex. These responses are summarized in Table 9.2.

To simplify this material, *it is best to study how specific hormone responses and functions are involved in key adaptations to exercise stress*;

1. Energy Metabolism

2. Fluid Balance

3. Vascular Hemodynamics

4. Protein Synthesis and Reproductive Function

Table 9.2: Summary of hormones involved in the acute adaptation to exercise. (simplification)

Gland/Hormones	Stimulant for Release	Target Tissue	Response
Cellular Energy Metabolism			
Adrenal Medulla			
Epinephrine	↑ Stress or Exercise Intensity, Hypotension	Skeletal muscle	↑ glycogenolysis
Norepinephrine	↑ Stress or Exercise Intensity, Hypoglycemia	Adipose tissue, Liver	↑ Lipolysis, ↑ HR, ↑ glycogenolysis, ↑stroke volume, ↑ vascular resistance

Table 9.2: Summary of hormones involved in the acute adaptation to exercise, cont'd. (simplification)

Gland/Hormones	Stimulant for Release	Target Tissue	Response
Fuel Mobilization			
Anterior Pituitary			
GH	Exercise Hypoglycemia	Skeletal muscle, Adipose tissue, Liver	FFA mobilization, ↑ Gluconeogenesis, ↓ Glucose uptake
Adrenal Cortex			
Cortisol	↑ ACTH, ↑ Exercise Intensity or Duration	Skeletal muscle, Adipose tissue, Liver	↑ Gluconeogenesis, ↑ Protein synthesis, ↓ Glucose uptake

Table 9.2: Summary of hormones involved in the acute adaptation to exercise, cont'd. (simplification)

Gland/Hormones	Stimulant for Release	Target Tissue	Response
Fuel Mobilization, cont'd.			
Pancreas			
Insulin	Hyperglycemia, ↑ blood amino acids	Skeletal muscle, Adipose tissue	↑ uptake of Glucose, Amino acids, FFA
Glucagon	Hypoglycemia, ↓ blood amino acids, Prolonged exercise	Liver	↑ Gluconeogenesis

Table 9.2: Summary of hormones involved in the acute adaptation to exercise, cont'd. (simplification)

Gland/Hormones	Stimulant for Release	Target Tissue	Response
Thyroid			
Triiodthyronine (T3) and Thyroxine (T4)	↓ T3 and T4	All	↑ Metabolic rate, GH, serum FFA, amino acids
Testes			
Testosterone	↑ FSH, LH Exercise (?)	Skeletal muscle, Testes, bone	↑ Protein synthesis, Sperm production, Sex drive
Ovaries			
Estrogen	↑ FSH, LH, Exercise intensity and duration	Skeletal muscle, Adipose tissue	↓ Glucose uptake, ↑ Fat oxidation, ↓ Glycogenolysis (?)

Table 9.2: Summary of hormones involved in the acute adaptation to exercise, cont'd. (simplification)

Gland/Hormones	Stimulant for Release	Target Tissue	Response
Fluid balance			
Posterior Pituitary			
ADH	↑ Plasma osmolality	Kidneys	↑ Water reabsorption
Kidneys			
Renin	↓ Urine flow	Blood	Angiotensinogen to angiotensin I
Adrenal Cortex			
Aldosterone	Angiotensin II	Kidneys	↑ Na reabsorption, ↑ Water reabsorption
Heart			
ANP	Hyperhydration	Pituitary	↓ ADH

Table 9.2: Summary of hormones involved in the acute adaptation to exercise, cont'd. (simplification)

Gland/Hormones	Stimulant for Release	Target Tissue	Response
Vascular hemodynamics			
Adrenal medulla			
Norepinephrine	Stress, Hypotenision, ↑ Exercise	Vascular smooth muscle	Vasoconstriction
Epinephrine	Stress, Hypoglycemia, ↑ Exercise	Vascular smooth muscle	Vasoconstriction
Posterior Pituitary			
ADH	↑ Plasma osmolality	Vascular smooth muscle	Vasoconstriction

Table 9.2: Summary of hormones involved in the acute adaptation to exercise, cont'd. (simplification)

Gland/Hormones	Stimulant for Release	Target Tissue	Response
Vascular hemodynamics, cont'd			
Endothelium			
Endothelin (ET)	Tissue Damage (?)	Local vasculature (?)	Vasoconstriction
Nitric Oxide (NO or EDRF)	?	Local vasculature (?)	Vasodilation

---

Table 9.2: Summary of hormones involved in the acute adaptation to exercise, cont'd. (simplification)

Gland/Hormones	Stimulant for Release	Target Tissue	Response
Muscle repair/hypertrophy			
Anterior Pituitary			
GH	↑ Stress, ↑ Exercise	Mainly bone	Growth
Various cells			
IGF-1	↑ GH	Most cells	Growth
Testes			
Testosterone	↑ Stress, ↑ Exercise	Skeletal muscle	↑ Protein synthesis

---

Exercise and Non-Insulin Dependent (Type II) Diabetes

Diabetes is a condition characterized by a decreased ability of cells to take up glucose, resulting in *hyperglycemia*. A sustained hyperglycemia can eventually *cause peripheral nerve damage*, which in turn can lead to *limb amputation* and *blindness*.

Type I - when there is an inability to produce insulin
(10% incidence)

Type II a) decreased ability to secrete insulin

b) decreased ability for cells to respond to insulin
(90% incidence)

Exercise training helps the Type II diabetic most by,

❖ ↑ GLUT4 sarcolemmal protein density

❖ ↑ insulin independent *glucose uptake* by skeletal muscle (acute and long term)

❖ reducing body fat (best in combination with a sound diet)

❖ ↑ in lean body mass

❖ ↑ insulin sensitivity

_____

_____

_____

_____

_____

_____

_____

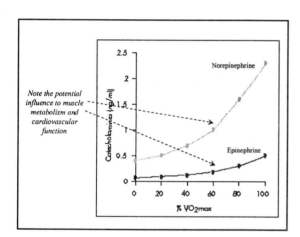

_____

_____

_____

_____

_____

_____

_____

_____

_____

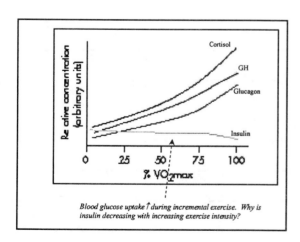

_____

_____

_____

_____

_____

_____

_____

_____

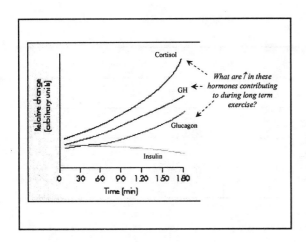

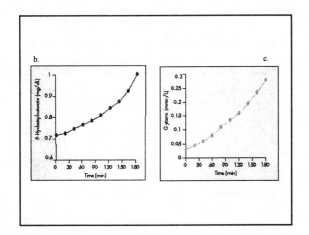

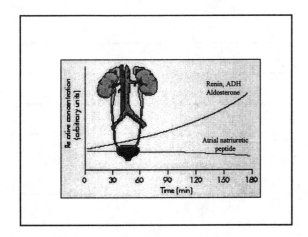

Exercise and the Control of Blood Pressure

In regulating vascular smooth muscle and also fluid balance, hormones are also very important in the long regulation of blood pressure.

Adjustment of *vasodilation* and *vasoconstriction* of arterioles modifies *vascular resistance* and blood pressure.

Adjustment of body hydration, alters *blood volume*, which in turn also alters *vascular resistance* and modifies blood pressure.

_____

_____

_____

_____

_____

_____

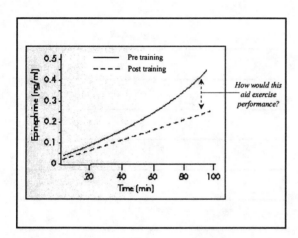

How would this aid exercise performance?

_____

_____

_____

_____

_____

_____

_____

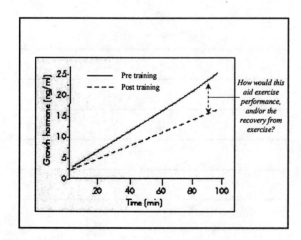

How would this aid exercise performance, and/or the recovery from exercise?

_____

_____

_____

_____

_____

_____

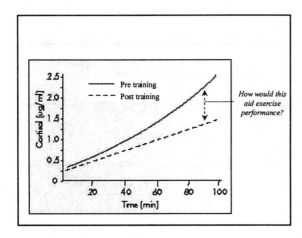

How would this aid exercise performance?

Reproductive Hormones

Amenorrhea - the absence of menstruation in women who should menstruate.

Athletic amenorrhea - when the cause of the amenorrhea is directly associated with exercise/training.

What causes athletic amenorrhea?

Negative feedback to the hypothalmus from
- ↑ β-endorphins
- ↑ catecholamines
- ↑ cortisol

The anterior pituitary is then prevented from releasing LH and FSH, which prevents the development of the follicle and release of estrogen and progesterone.

PART 3

Methods to Improve Exercise Performance

Chapter 10

Training For Sport and Performance

Fitness and Training

Training - the organized sequence of exercise that stimulates adaptations in anatomy and physiology. These adaptations are termed *training adaptations*, or *chronic adaptations*

Fitness - a general term that actually contains many components:

cardiorespiratory endurance   muscular endurance

muscular strength   muscular power

flexibility   body composition

emotional/psychological qualities

Principles of Training

Specificity

Training should be based on the specific demands/needs of the sport/event. The better one can understand these demands/needs, the more likely one can develop a suitable training program.

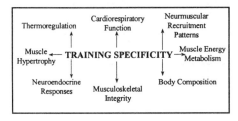

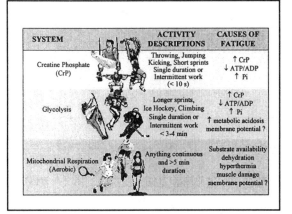

Research Findings

VO₂max

➤ VO_2max is largest in the trained exercise mode for well-trained individuals

➤ There is partial transfer in VO_2max improvement between run and cycle training

Lactate Threshold

➤ For well trained individuals, the LT and VT are more sensitive indices of training improvement that VO_2max

➤ There is partial transfer in LT improvement between run and cycle training

Intense Exercise and Weight Lifting

➤ long distance running decreases muscle power

➤ Research of training using isokinetic muscle contractions indicates that the velocity of contraction is an important component of training specificity

➤ Little is known of how to time strength/power and endurance training so that the benefits of each are maximized

Cross Training

➤ Defined as training in different modes of exercise

➤ When used correctly, cross training can improve the quality of training by - ↑ *stimulus for adaptation, maintaining muscle power,* and *preventing injuries*

Overload and Overtraining

Overload is a principle based on the need to train above a stimulus threshold for the development of chronic training adaptations

Overtaining is a condition that occurs when an athlete has trained too hard or for durations that are too long to allow full recovery. A decrease in performance remains the most sensitive gauge of overtraining.

The nature of the overload stimulus depends on;

• *Exercise intensity*	• *Recovery duration*
• *Exercise duration*	• *Type of exercise*
• *Frequency of exercise sessions*	• *Initial level of fitness*

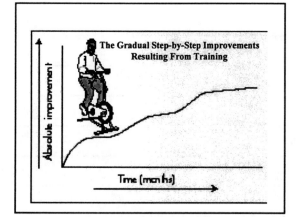

The Gradual Step-by-Step Improvements Resulting From Training

Absolute improvement

Time (months)

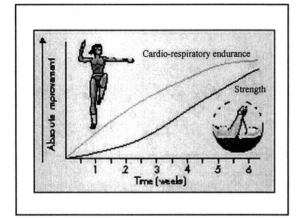

Additional symptoms of overtraining

- ↳ ↑ Resting heart rate
- ↳ ↓ Body weight
- ↳ ↓ Appetite
- ↳ Muscle soreness that is retained > 24 hrs
- ↳ ↑ Serum LDH and CK activity
- ↳ Worse running economy and ↑ submaximal HR
- ↳ ↑ Incidence of illness (colds, flu, etc.)
- ↳ ↑ Constipation or diarrhea
- ↳ ↓ Performance
- ↳ Lack of desire to train or compete

The Taper

Involves a period of reduced training (days to several weeks) prior to athletic competition. Research shows that a correct taper,

- ✖ does not ↓ VO_2max
- ✖ ↑ muscle power
- ✖ ↑ performance

Reversibility and Detraining can occur if the training stimulus is completely removed. Bed rest can ↓ VO2max by 27% in 20 days

DETRAINING

Other
Loss of heat acclimation

Body composition
↑ Body fat
↓ Lean body mass
↑ Body weight

Pulmonary Function
↓ Respiratory muscle strength & endurance

Cardiovascular function
↓ Red blood cell mass
↓ End diastolic volume
↓ Plasma volume

Skeletal muscle
↓ Mitochondrial density
↓ Capillary density
↓ Muscular strength

Retraining concerns whether previously trained individuals have a more rapid rate of adaptation after a return to training. *This concept is not supported by research.*

Methods of Training

Cadiorespiratory and Muscular Endurance

- ↗ Continuous
- ↗ Interval
- ↗ Fartlek

Muscular Strength and Hypertrophy

- ✦ *Repetitions, Sets, Recovery*
- ✦ *Circuit Training*
- ✦ *Periodization*
- ✦ *Pyramid System*
- ✦ *Split Routine System*
- ✦ *Eccentric Loading*
- ✦ *Plyometric Training*
- ✦ *Super Set System*

Chapter 11

Resistance Exercise and Muscular Strength

Basic Definitions:

Resistance Exercise - muscle contractions performed against resistance (load).

Strength - greatest force than can be applied for a given contraction velocity.

Maximal Voluntary Contraction (MVC) - strength measured during an isometric contraction.

1 RM – One repetition maximum = maximum weight that can be lifted once

---

Types of Contractions:

Isometric – tension development with no change in muscle length.

Dynamic - tension development with a change in muscle length.

  concentric – muscle shortens during contraction

  eccentric – muscle lengthens during contraction

  isokinetic – muscle contraction at a fixed velocity

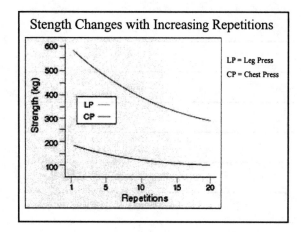

Stength Changes with Increasing Repetitions

LP = Leg Press
CP = Chest Press

Chapter 12

Nutrition and Exercise

Exercise Nutrition

- **Pre-exercise Nutrition**
  Recommended quantities of Macronutrients
  Estimating Fluid Requirements
  Pre-exercise Meal

- **Nutrition During Exercise**
  CHO intake
  Hydration

- **Post Exercise Nutrition**
  Glycogen replenishment
  Rehydration

Nutrition

Nutrients - molecules needed by cells to function optimally.

Micronutrients - small nutrients that are not catabolized to release free energy during metabolism.

Macronutrients - nutrients that can be catabolized during metabolism.

Micronutrients

The micronutrients consists of,
- vitamins
- minerals *a.k.a. trace elements*

The quantity of micronutrients needed each day are established in the "Recommended Daily Allowances (RDA's)

Macronutrients

The macronutrients consists of,

- carbohydrates   • lipids   • proteins

A macronutrient RDA only exists for protein,
0.8 - 1.2 g protein / kg body mass

It is recommended that a normal balanced diet should have,
carbohydrate Kcals = 60% total
lipid Kcals   = 30% total
= 10% saturated + 10% monounsaturated + 10% polyunsaturated
protein Kcals   = 10% total

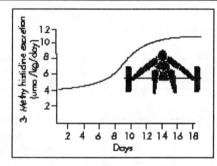

*Due to ↑ protein catabolism and ↑ post-exercise synthesis, the
RDA for protein may increase to 1.2 - 2 g/kg/day, depending on
the exercise conditions*

Water - also a very important nutrient, with a base recommendation
of ~ *2.5 L/day.*   Conversion: 1 cup (8oz.) = 240 mL

Estimating Fluid Needs (healthy individuals)

*Moderate to profuse sweating can increase the following
fluid requirements by 500 - 1000 mL or more!*

I. Body Weight
100 mL/kg/24 hr   for first 0 - 10 kg
50 mL/kg/24 hr   for next 11 - 20 kg
20 mL/kg/24 hr   for additional weight over 20 kg

Example: 60 kg Individual
(100 mL x 10) + (50 mL x 10) + (20 mL x 40) = **2300mL**

Estimating Fluid Needs, cont.

II. 35 mL per kg body weight per day (range of 30 - 50 mL)

Example: 60 kg Female
35 mL x 60 kg = **2100 mL**

III. One mL per calorie consumed

Example: 2000 kcal/day diet
1 mL x 2000 kcal = **2000 mL**

Handbook of Dietetic Formulas: Nutrition Services and Clinical Dietetics, 1st ed.

Major micronutrients and macronutrients and their functions that support exercise.

NUTRIENT	FUNCTIONS	SOURCES
MICRONUTRIENTS		
VITAMINS		
WATER SOLUBLE		
Thiamine (B1)	coenzyme	Pork, organ meats, whole grains, legumes
Riboflavin (B2)	Component of FAD^+ and FMN	Most foods
Niacin	Component of NAD^+ and $NADP^+$	Liver, lean meats, grains, legumes
Pyridoxine (B6)	coenzyme	Meats, vegetables, whole grains
Pantothenic acid	Component of coenzyme A	Most foods

Major micronutrients and macronutrients, cont'd

NUTRIENT	FUNCTIONS	SOURCES
Folacin	Coenzyme	Legumes, green vegetables, whole wheat
Cobalamin (B12)	Coenzyme	Muscle meat, eggs, dairy products
Biotin	Coenzyme	Meats, vegetables, legumes
Ascorbic acid (C)	Maintains connective tissue Immune protection	Citrus fruits, tomatoes, green peppers
FAT SOLUBLE		
β-carotene (provitamin A) *Retinol (A)*	Sight; component of rhodopsin Maintains tissues	Milk, butter, cheese
Cholecalciferol (D)	Bone growth Ca^{++} absorption	Cod liver oil, eggs, dairy products

Major micronutrients and macronutrients, cont'd

NUTRIENT	FUNCTIONS	SOURCES
Tocopherol (E)	Anti-oxidant	Seeds, green leafy vegetables, margarine
Phylloquinone (K)	Blood clotting	Green leafy vegetables, cereals, fruits, meat
MAJOR MINERALS		
Calcium (Ca^{++})	Bone and tooth formation, muscle contraction, action potentials	Milk, cheese, dark green vegetables
Phosphorus (PO_3^-)	Bone and tooth formation, acid-base, chemical energy	Milk, cheese, yogurt, meat, poultry, grains, fish
Potassium (K^+)	Action potential, acid-base, water balance	Leafy vegetables, cantaloupe, lima beans, potatoes, milk, meat

---

Major micronutrients and macronutrients, cont'd

NUTRIENT	FUNCTIONS	SOURCES
Sulphur (S)	Aid-base, liver function	Proteins, dried foods
Sodium (Na^+)	Action potential, acid-base, osmolality, body waterbalance	Fruits, vegetables, table salt
Chlorine (Cl)	Membrane potential, fluid balance	Fruits, vegetables, table salt
Magnesium (Mg^{2+})	Enzyme cofactor	Whole grains, green leafy vegetables
MINOR MINERALS		
Iron (Fe)	Components of hemoglobin, myoglobin, cytochromes	Eggs, lean meats, legumes, whole grains, green leafy vegetables

---

Major micronutrients and macronutrients, cont'd

NUTRIENT	FUNCTIONS	SOURCES
Flourine (F)	Bone and teeth structure	Water, seafood
Zinc (Zn)	Component of enzymes	Most foods
Copper (Cu)	Component of enzymes	Meat, water
Selenium (Se)	Functions with vitamin E	Seafood, meat, grains
Iodine (I)	Thyroid hormones	Marine fish and shellfish, dairyproducts, vegetales, iodized salt
Chromium (Cr)	Required for glycolysis	Legumes, cereals, organ meats
Molybdenum (Mo)	Enzyme cofactor	Fats, vegetable oils, meats, whole grains

Major micronutrients and macronutrients, cont'd

NUTRIENT	FUNCTIONS	SOURCES
MACRONUTRIENTS		
CARBOHYDRATES		
MONOSACCHARIDES		
Glucose	Tissue metabolism	Candies, fruit, processed food, soda
Fructose	Liver metabolism	Honey, corn, fruit
Galactose	Liver metabolism	Breast milk
DISACCHARIDES		
Sucrose	Energy metabolism	Table sugar, maple syrup, sugar cane
Lactose	No essential role	Dairy products
Maltose	No essential role	Formed during digestion

Major micronutrients and macronutrients, cont'd

NUTRIENT	FUNCTIONS	SOURCES
POLYSACCHARIDES		
Statch	Tissue metabolism	Candies, fruit, processed food, soda
Fiber	Liver metabolism	Honey, corn, fruit
LIPIDS		
Cholesterol	Cell membranes, steroid hormones	Beef, liver, eggs, butter, shrimp
Triglycerides and fatty acids	Energy metabolism, insulation, organ protection	Meats, oils, nuts, cheese, whole milk and other dairy products
Omega-3-fatty acids	May ↓ blood choleserol and atheroslerosis	Cold water fish oils
Saturated fat	?	Coconut oil, butter, cream, animal fat

Major micronutrients and macronutrients, cont'd

NUTRIENT	FUNCTIONS	SOURCES
Monounsaturated fat	?	Olives, almonds, avocados, peanuts
Polyunsaturated fat	?	Safflower and sunflower oil, sesame seeds
PROTEIN		
Complete	Cell maintenance, structure and repair, immune function	Meat, poultry, eggs, cheese, fish, milk
Incomplete	Cell maintenance, structure and repair, immune function	Legumes, cereal, seeds, leafy vegetables
WATER		Drinking water, juices, sodas, fruits, vegetables

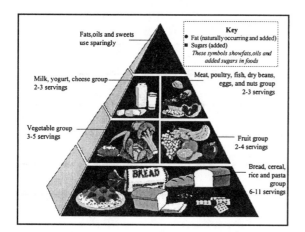

Key
- Fat (naturally occurring and added)
- Sugars (added)

These symbols show fats, oils and added sugars in foods

Fats, oils and sweets use sparingly

Milk, yogurt, cheese group 2-3 servings

Meat, poultry, fish, dry beans, eggs, and nuts group 2-3 servings

Vegetable group 3-5 servings

Fruit group 2-4 servings

Bread, cereal, rice and pasta group 6-11 servings

Recommended Serving Sizes

Milk	1 cup
Yogurt	1 cup
Cheese	1 oz
Eggs	1
Beans/peas	1/2 cup
Peanut Butter	2 tbsp
Whole fruit (orange, apple)	1
Grapefruit (1/2) Cantaloupe (1/3)	
Choppped raw vegetables	1/2 cup
Leafy green vegetables	1 cup
Bread	1 slice
Dry Cereal	1 oz or 3/4 cup

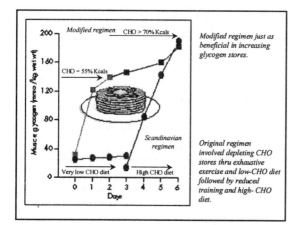

Modified regimen just as beneficial in increasing glycogen stores.

Original regimen involved depleting CHO stores thru exhaustive exercise and low-CHO diet followed by reduced training and high-CHO diet.

Recommendations for increasing muscle glycogen stores in the days before prolonged exercise.

1. Plan to taper at least 1 week before the event.

2. In the final week, train as planned and eat your typical diet during the first 3 days.

3. For the 3 days prior to event, increase the carbohydrate content of the diet to more than 10 g/kg body weight/day.

Example: 60 kg individual on typical 3000 kcal, 60% CHO diet
3000 kcal x .60 = 1800 kcal CHO ÷ 4 kcal/g = 450 g CHO
450 g ÷ 60 kg = 7.5 g CHO / kg of BW
10 g CHO x 60 kg BW = 600 g CHO
600 g x 4 kcal/g = 2400 kcal CHO
which is an increase to 80% CHO diet

It is recommended for athletes expending large amounts of calories due to training, that the % of calories from carbohydrate be increased and the % of calories from fat be decreased.

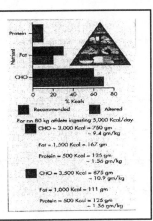

Rebound Hypoglycemia

↑ insulin levels and ↑ uptake of glucose from exercising muscle leads to rapid decline in blood glucose levels.

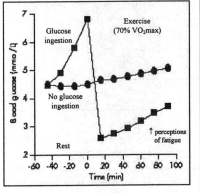

Timing Carbohydrate Ingestion Prior to Exercise

• Large meal up to 6 hours prior to competition.

• Smaller meals containing less than 100 g of CHO can be ingested up to 45 minutes before exercise. (tops off glycogen stores)

• Carbohydrate can be ingested just prior to exercise (within 15 minutes). Does not allow adequate time for insulin levels to increase and exercise then depresses insulin release.

• Avoid high fat meals prior to exercise to reduce gastric-intestinal stress and discomfort.

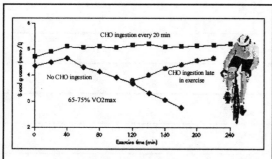

Carbohydrate ingestion late in exercise produces similar responses to ingestion of carbohydrate throughout the exercise session. *Interpreted as CHO supplementing blood glucose, not sparing muscle glycogen.*

Gastric emptying research tells us:

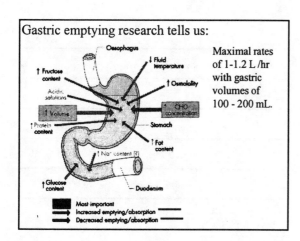

Maximal rates of 1-1.2 L /hr with gastric volumes of 100 - 200 mL.

> Gastric emptying is slowed when drinks contain ↑ CHO, ↑ osmolality, ↑ protein/amino acids, ↓ pH.

> The intestinal absorption of water is increased when CHO is present.

> Electrolyte loss from the body is minimal and does not warrant replacement during exercise.

> There is wide individual variability in drink tolerance.

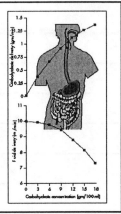

Electrolytes in plasma and sweat and electrolyte loss during severe (> 5%) exercise-induced dehydration

Electrolyte	Plasma (mEq/L)	Sweat (mEq/L)	Losses (mEq)
Na^+	140	40-60	155
K^+	4	4-5	16
Cl^-	101	30-50	137
Mg^{++}	1.5	1.5-5	13
Osmolality	302	80-195	

Liquid Carbohydrate Ingestion

> Suited for long duration (> 60 min) exercise where a glucose source is needed to support blood glucose

> Need at least 45 g/CHO/Hr

> Drink of 60 g CHO/L would require at least 750 mL/Hr

> During hot and humid conditions, a lower [CHO] drink would allow greater volumes to be ingested.

> Most people can not ingest more than 1.2 L/Hr

> CHO should be mostly glucose

Nutrient and electrolyte content of commercial drinks.

DRINK	CHO (g/100 mL)	Na+ (mEq/L)	K+ (mEq/L)	Caffeine (mg/L)	Osmolality (mOsmol/kg)
10K	6.3	52	26		350
Coca-Cola	10.7	2	0	136.8	554
Cranberry juice	10-15	2	7		890
Dioralyte	1.6	60	20		?
Exceed	6.0	21	3		250
Gatorade	6.0	21	3		280
Isostar	7.6	24	4		305
Orange juice	11.8	0.5	58		690
Sprite	10.2	5	0		695
Water	0	trace	trace		0-20

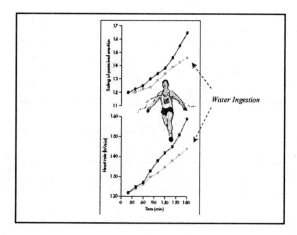

Water Ingestion

Muscle Glycogen Synthesis

Muscle glycogen is synthesized very slowly. The rate of synthesis differs depending on the prior exercise conditions,

after low intensity exercise - 7-9 mmol/kg/Hr

after high intensity exercise - ~ 15 mmol/kg/Hr

Muscle glycogen synthesis is optimized when,

✓ there has been *no exercise-induced muscle damage*

✓ *recovery is passive*

✓ at least *0.7 g CHO/kg/Hr is ingested*

✓ ingestion occurs *as soon after exercise* as possible

✓ *glucose should be the predominant CHO* and the source food should have a high glycemic index

Glycemic Index

Relative index for comparing the blood glucose response from the ingestion of different foods. In general, the more complex the carbohydrate, and the more fat, protein and fiber in the food, the lower is the glycemic index.

FOOD ITEM	GLYCEMIC INDEX
Cornflakes	121
Instant mashed potatoes	120
Whole wheat bread	100
Baked beans	70
Skim milk	46
White pasta (boiled)	45
Lentils (boiled)	36

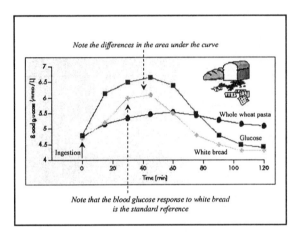

Note the differences in the area under the curve

Note that the blood glucose response to white bread is the standard reference

Post-exercise Nutrition

Rehydration

As previously indicated, it is difficult to prevent dehydration during prolonged exercise. Rehydration is improved when,

✳ a CHO-electrolyte solution is ingested

✳ volume ingested > 1.5 x body weight loss

✳ glycerol is added to the drink

Severe dehydration (> 4% body weight loss) can require more than 24 Hrs for complete rehydration

Chapter 13

Ergogenic Aids

Ergogenic is defined as "tending to increase work"

An **ergogenic aid** is defined as ".. *A physical, mechanical, nutritional, psychological, or pharmacological substance or treatment that either directly improves physiological variables associated with exercise performance or removes subjective restraints which may limit physiological capacity"*

Some examples of ergogenic aids are;

Warm-up	Caffeine ingestion	Carbohydrate ingestion
Liquid ingestion	Glycerol ingestion	Phosphate ingestion
NaHCO$_3^-$ ingestion	Creatine ingestion	Blood doping
Erythropoietin	Growth hormone	Testosterone

Warm-up

Benefits of warm-up

BENEFIT	Verified by Research
Submaximal Exercise	
Muscle temperature	Yes
Muscle blood flow	Yes
Oxygen deficit	Yes
Neuromuscular function	No
Lipid catabolism	Yes
Carbohydrate metabolism	Yes
Muscle glycogen sparing	No
Risk of musculoskeletal injury ..	No

Cont'd.

BENEFIT	Verified by Research
Intense Exercise	
↑ *Neuromuscular function*	Yes
↑ *Lipid catabolism*	No
↓ *Carbohydrate metabolism*	No
Improved acid base balance	Yes
↓ *Oxygen deficit*	Yes
Muscle glycogen sparing	No
↓ *Risk of musculoskeletal injury*	No

Nutritional Ergogenic Aids

- ◀ Caffeine
- ◀ Glycerol
- ◀ Carnitine
- ◀ Phosphate
- ◀ Sodium Bicarbonate
- ◀ Dichloroacetate
- ◀ Creatine
- ◀ Branched chain amino acids

Caffeine

▸ The most highly consumed drug in North America and Europe

▸ IOC initially banned caffeine in 1962, then removed from list in 1972

▸ Today, urinary caffeine > 12 mg/L is an IOC infringement

▸ This urinary level requires > 13.5 mg/kg caffeine, where 1 cup coffee provides 80 mg   *Assume 75 kg body mass*

IOC banned dosage	*Ergogenic benefit*
1012 mg/80 = 12.7 cups	330 mg/80 = 4.1 cups

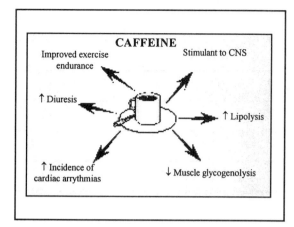

CAFFEINE

Improved exercise endurance

Stimulant to CNS

↑ Diuresis

↑ Lipolysis

↑ Incidence of cardiac arrythmias

↓ Muscle glycogenolysis

Glycerol

Ingestion of ~1.2 g glycerol/kg body mass with sufficient volumes of water (26 mL/kg) can induce an increase in hydration, termed *hyperhydration*.

Glycerol hyperhydration procedure

Time (min)	Ingestion	Comment
0	5 mL/kg of 20% glycerol	Glycerol dose = 1.0 g/kg
30	5 mL/kg water	
45	5 mL/kg water	
60	1 mL/kg of 20% glycerol	Glycerol dose = 0.2 g/kg
90	5 mL/kg water	
150		Start Exercise

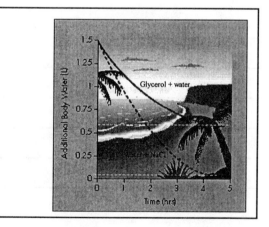

Carnitine

Molecule that transports fatty acids into mitochondria. Research indicates that carnitine provides no ergogenic benefit.

Phosphate

Some evidence for increased VO_2max and VT.

Sodium Bicarbonate

Increases blood bicarbonate and buffering potential. Increases performance during intense intermittent exercise.

Creatine

● Creatine is the main component of creatine phosphate. Creatine is found in meat and fish, but is also able to be synthesized in the body.

● Dietary supplementation of creatine of at least 15 g/day for 2-7 days can increase muscle CrP and free Cr.

● The physiological benefits of creatine ingestion are summarized in Figure 12.3

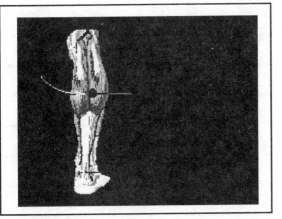

Branched Chain Amino Acids

The main BCAA's are leucine, isoleucine and valine. These amino acids decrease the ability for tryptophan to cross the blood brain barrier, impeding the formation of seratonin and the perception of fatigue (central fatigue).

Other Ergogenic Aids
Pure Oxygen Inhalation

▸ This procedure can raise blood PaO_2 from 104 mmHg at sea level to ~600 mmHg.

▸ This raises the blood oxygen content;

104 x 0.03 mL/L/mmHg = 3.12 mL/L

600 x 0.03 mL/L/mmHg = 18 mL/L

18 - 3.12 = **14.88** mL/L

▸ The raised blood O_2 content can increase VO_2max. However, there is no evidence that breathing pure oxygen aids recovery.

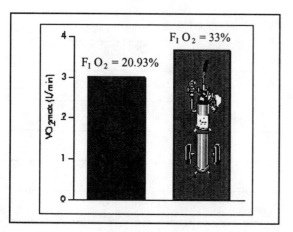

Erythropoietin (EPO)

► A hormone that is mainly produced in the kidney in response to hypoxia, anemia, and blood loss.

► EPO stimulates increased red blood cell production (erythropoiesis).

► EPO is widely used by elite endurance athletes, but has caused deaths due to excessive increases in blood viscosity and organ damage.

_____

_____

_____

_____

_____

_____

Blood Doping

⚴ The removal of 1-4 units of blood, storage of the blood for 4-8 weeks, and the reinfusion of the red blood cells.

⚴ Reinfusion usually occurs ~1 week prior to competition.

⚴ Blood doping can double the [Hb], but typically this causes too much of an increase in blood viscosity.

140 g/L x 1.34 mL/g x 0.98 = 148 mL/L
200 g/L x 1.34 mL/L x 0.98 = 263 mL/L
262 - 148 = **79** mL/L

_____

_____

_____

_____

_____

_____

⚴ Blood doping can increase VO_2max and improve endurance exercise performance.

Growth Hormone (GH)

▶ A natural glucoregulatory and anabolic hormone.

▶ GH use can -

  ⅄ ↑ muscle hypertrophy and strength
  ⅄ ↓ body fat
  ⅄ ↑ growth of flat bones
  ⅄ ↑ healing of musculo-skeletal injury

_____

_____

_____

_____

_____

_____

Anabolic-Androgenic Steroids

A family of hormones similar to testosterone.

Benefits are similar to GH, but include additional side-effects such as;

- hirsutism
- deepening of the voice
- acne
- aggressive behavior
- decrease in HDL cholesterol
- liver damage

Amphetamines

- Stimulants to the CNS, but far more potent than caffeine.
- Minimal research
- Increase risk for;
  - Over-exertion causing musculoskeletal injury
  - Cardiac arrhythmias
  - Hypertensive responses to exercise
  - Irritability
  - Paranoia

PART 4

Measurements of Fitness and Exercise Performance

Chapter 14

Measuring Endurance and Anaerobic Capacity

Metabolic Determinants of Physiological Capacities

✓ Certain activities/sports are reliant on high skeletal *muscle metabolic capacities*.

✓ If the metabolic demands and related physiology of given activities are known, then laboratory tests can be developed to *measure* or *be dependent on* that metabolic pathway.

✓ As will be shown, the metabolic needs of activities differ most in terms of their *exercise intensity/duration*.

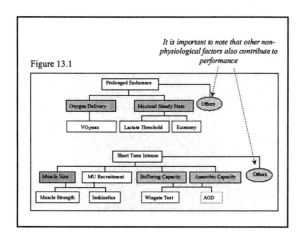

Figure 13.1

It is important to note that other non-physiological factors also contribute to performance

---

VO$_2$max

Traditionally, the maximal rate of oxygen consumption (VO$_2$max) is interpreted as a measure of the *maximal capacity of the body's cardiorespiratory function.*

The test of VO$_2$max is arguably the most performed test of human physiological function in exercise physiology.

Limitations

⌐ Additional variables are also important for performance

⌐ Does not explain who performs well among individuals with similar training

⌐ Requires sophisticated equipment

⌐ Difficult to measure a true maximal value is some people

Testing Procotols

The time constraints for the duration of a protocol suited to measure VO$_2$max necessitates the need to *tailor a protocol to suit a given individual.*

The steps to follow in determining a protocol are:

⊠ determine the subject's cardiorespiratory fitness and training status by interview, and estimate a workload at VO$_2$max.

⊠ Select suitable stage and total test durations.

⊠ Calculate the increment needed for each stage

Table 13.1: Criteria for a valid protocol to measure VO₂max

Criteria	Description
Protocol	
Test duration	8-12 min
Stage duration	Ramp, or 1-3 min
Intensity increment	Based on stage duration and cardiorespiratory fitness of subjects
Mode	Subject specific on the basis of training, disease states, and musculoskeletal concerns
Data Interpretation	
Criteria for max vs. peak	Plateau in VO₂ RER > 1.1 Hrmax < 10 b/min from predicted

Predicting Steady State VO₂

Steady state VO₂ can estimated using one of several equations (Table 13.2).

It is recommended that the *ACSM equations* be used for treadmill walking and running.

For cycle ergometry, the *equation of Latin* should be used.

Summary of submaximal VO₂ prediction equations (simplified)

Criteria	Equation
Treadmill Walking	
ACSM (mL/kg/min)	[0.1 (m/min)] + [(grade fraction) (m/min) (1.8)] + 3.5
Treadmill Running	
ACSM (mL/kg/min)	[0.2 (m/min)] + [(grade fraction) (m/min) (0.9)] + 3.5
Cycle Ergometry	
ACSM (mL/min)	[2 (kgm/min)] + [3.5 (wt,kg)]
Latin (mL/min)	[1.9 (kgm/min)] + [3.5 (wt,kg)] + 260

Predicting Cardiorespiratory and Muscular Endurance

VO_2max

VO_2max can be predicted from either *maximal* or *submaximal* exercise tests (Table 13.2).

Typically, submaximal tests are shorter in duration, and can used for more elderly subjects due to reduced risks for *musculoskeletal and cardiovascular injury*.

Maximal tests, despite the added time and effort required by the subject, are ***far more accurate***

Summary of prediction equations for VO_2max (simplified)

Criteria	Equation
Maximal Tests - Treadmill	
Bruce (mL/kg/min)	$6.7 - [2.82 (gender)] + [0.056 (time)]$
Foster (mL/kg/min)	$14.76 - [1.38 (time)] + 0.451 (time^2)] - [0.12 (time^3)]$
Maximal Tests – Cycle Ergometry	
Storer (mL/min)	
- male	$[10.51 (Wmax)] + [6.35 (wt, kg)] - [10.49 (age, yr)] + 519.3$
- female	$[9.39 (Wmax)] + [7.7 (wt, kg)] - [5.88 (age, yr)] + 136.7$

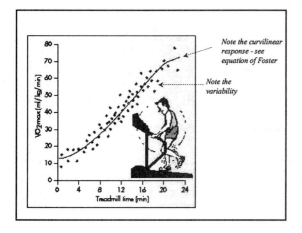

Note the curvilinear response - see equation of Foster

Note the variability

Submaximal Tests For Predicting Cardiorespiratory and Muscular Endurance

The most accurate and widely used protocols for estimating VO₂max from submaximal exercise are;

- ✗ ACSM equation (treadmill or cycle ergometer)
- ✗ YMCA cycle ergometer protocol
- ✗ Astrand-Rhyming nomogram
- ✗ Modifications of YMCA and Astrand-Rhyming nomogram

ACSM Equation

1. Complete steady state exercise for between 4-6 min for two exercise intensities. *(ideally between 60-85% HR-reserve)*

2. Measure the *steady state HR* for each condition.

3. Calculate VO_2 for each condition using the most accurate equation (Table 13.2).

4. Calculate the VO_2-HR slope (***b***)

5. Calculate HRmax (220 - age)

6. Calculate VO_2max

$$\boldsymbol{b} = (\text{B}VO_2 - \text{A}VO_2) / (\text{BHR} - \text{AHR})$$

$$\textbf{VO}_\textbf{2}\textbf{max} = \text{B}VO_2 + [\boldsymbol{b}\,(\text{HRmax} - \text{BHR})]$$

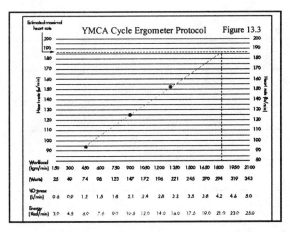

YMCA Cycle Ergometer Protocol   Figure 13.3

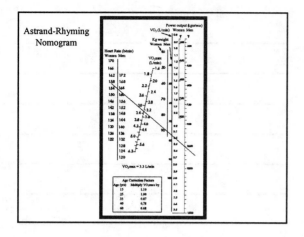

Astrand-Rhyming Nomogram

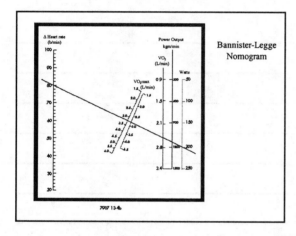

Bannister-Legge Nomogram

Lactate and Ventilatory Thresholds

The exercise intensity at the lactate threshold (LT) or ventilatory threshold (VT) provides the *best measurement that can predict athletic performance* in middle to long distance (duration) events.

There are currently *no universally accepted guidelines for measuring the LT*, and *several methods exist* for documenting a threshold change in blood lactate.

More concrete guidelines exist for the VT, with one of two methods being acceptable in research (see Figure 8.10):

- ventilatory equivalents (V_E/VO_2 vs VO_2)
- V-Slope (VCO_2 vs VO_2)

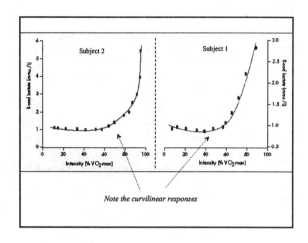

Note the curvilinear responses

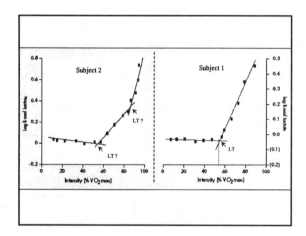

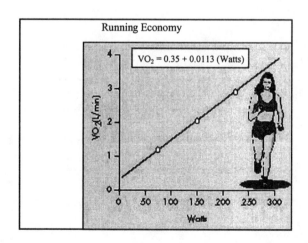

Running Economy

$VO_2 = 0.35 + 0.0113 \text{ (Watts)}$

Other Tests of Cardiorespiratory and Muscular Endurance

VO$_2$ Kinetics

The more rapid the increase in VO$_2$ during a rest-exercise transition, the greater the cardiorespiratory and muscular endurance of the subject.

The increase in VO$_2$ to steady state is represented by a monoexponential equation:

$$VO_2 = A\ (1 - e^{-Bx}) + E$$

A = magnitude of change, e = natural log base, B = rate constant, E = beginning VO$_2$, x = time

see Figures 6.9 and 6.13

Heart Rate Threshold

Heart rate does not increase in a linear manner to VO$_2$max in all individuals. The exercise intensity *where HR-VO$_2$ deviates from linearity* has been termed the **heart rate threshold** (HRT or *fc*).

The *fc* has been shown to coincide with the LT, but additional studies have not confirmed this association. Furthermore, a *fc* may only occur in ~50% of healthy individuals.

See Figure 7.7

Predicting Maximal Muscle Power and Anaerobic Capacity

The muscles' capacity for non-mitochondrial (*anaerobic*) ATP regeneration is impossible to measure accurately. Due to this, several laboratory tests have been developed that rely heavily on anaerobic ATP regeneration, or indirectly provide a measure of the anaerobic capacity.

Short-Term Tests	Intermediate-Term Tests
Sargeant's Jump and Reach	Wingate Test
Margaria Power Test	Isokinetic Tests
	Muscle Metabolite Accumulation
	Accumulated Oxygen Deficit

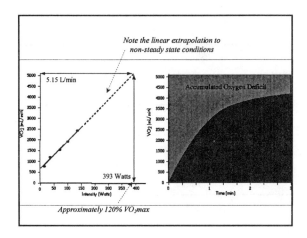

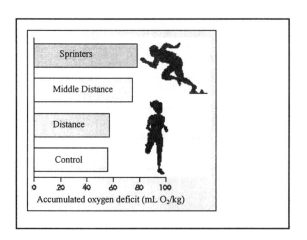

Chapter 15

Estimating Body Composition

What is Body Composition?

Refers to the relative amounts of the different compounds in the body

Why Study Body Composition?

- Overweight vs. Over fat vs. Obesity
- Risk for various diseases
- Monitor change from an intervention
- Some job requirements involve body composition standards
- Athletic/sports prowess

Body Mass Index (BMI)

The ratio of mass to height^2

BMI = body mass (kg) / body height (m)^2

for example

BMI = 80 (kg) / 1.7^2 (m) = 27.68 kg/m^2

BMI < 20.0 is considered underweight (see Table 15.2)

A BMI > 30 is associated with greater prevalence of mortality from heart disease, cancer, and diabetes

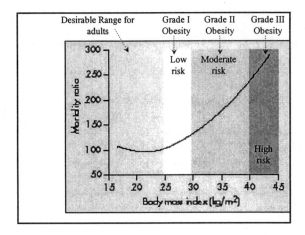

Understanding Body Fat

Fat Body Mass (FBM)- includes both essential and storage fat

Essential Fat - found in bone marrow, the brain and spinal cord, muscles, and other internal organs.

     Approximates 3% of total body weight for men

     Approximates 3% of total body weight for women

Storage Fat - 99% is yellow (adipose tissue) fat

     1% is brown fat

Lean Body Mass (LBM) - includes fat free body mass and essential fat

Fat Free Body Mass (FFBM) - all body tissue excluding lipid and fat. However, LBM is used synonymously.

Ideal Weight

The weight that would result from desired values for FBM and FFBM

for example

Fat weight = current weight (kg) x (% fat/100)

Lean Body Mass = current weight (kg) - fat weight

Ideal weight = LBM / [1 - (% fat desired / 100)]

Desirable fat loss = current weight - ideal body weight

The Two-Component System of Body Composition

This is the historical/traditional system for body composition assessment and quantification.

- Lean Body Mass (more accurately the FFBM)

- Fat Body Mass

The two component system has the following assumptions:

1. Fat density = 0.90 g/mL at 37°C

2. LBM density = 1.10 g/mL at 37°C

3. All individuals have the above mass densities

4. LBM is 73.8% water, 19.4% protein, and 6.8% mineral

The Compartmental Models of Body Composition

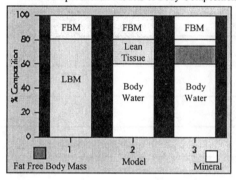

Methods for the Two Component Model

⇔ Hydrodensitometry

⇔ Air-displacement plethysmography (BodPod™)

Hydrodensitometry
(underwater weighing or hydrostatic weighing)
Has been termed the "gold standard" of body composition assessment. However, inadequacies of the assumptions can cause errors as large as ±4% fat.

This method is based on *Archimedes' principle*, where a person's weight underwater is used to calculate body volume. Body density is then calculated, and specific equations are used that convert body density into %fat.

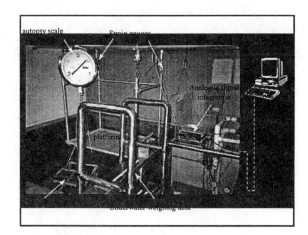

Body Density (Db) = body mass (g) / body volume (mL)

$$Db = Wa / \{[(Wa - Ww) / Dw] - (RV + 100 \, mL)\}$$

where;
    Db = body density (g/mL)

    Wa = body mass out of water

    Ww = body mass underwater

    Dw = density of water (g/mL)

    RV = residual lung volume (mL)

Siri Equation - % body fat = $[(4.95 / Db) - 4.50] \times 100$

Brozek Equation - % body fat = $[(4.57 / Db) - 4.142] \times 100$

Alternative equations to those of Siri and Brozek

Age	Gender	% Body Fat	D_{FFB}
15-16	M	$[(5.03 / Db) - 4.59] \times 100$	1.0960
	F	$[(5.07 / Db) - 4.64] \times 100$	1.0940
17-19	M	$[(4.98 / Db) - 4.53] \times 100$	1.0985
	F	$[(5.05 / Db) - 4.62] \times 100$	1.0950
20-50	M	$[(4.95 / Db) - 4.50] \times 100$	1.1000
	F	$[(5.03 / Db) - 4.59] \times 100$	1.0960

Other Methods

- Skinfolds

- Dual X-Ray Absorptiometry (DEXA)

- Bioelectrical Impedance

- Near-Infrared Interactance

_____

_____

_____

_____

_____

_____

_____

PART 5

Special Topics Within Exercise Physiology

Chapter 16

Growth, Development, Aging and Exercise

Exercise and Children

Children are not small adults in how they respond to exercise. Nevertheless, many of the physiological responses to exercise are similar between children and adults.

Research tells us:

♥ Too many children do not engage in enough *vigorous* physical activity

♥ Participation in physical activity declines as age increases during school years

♥ Daily *enrolment in physical education* classes dropped from 42 to 25% among high school students between 1991-1995

♥ Children need help to develop appropriate exercise habits

Health and Fitness of Children

Beginning in the 1950's and early 1960's, several organizations began surveying youth fitness in the United States.

AAHPER

Institute For Aerobics Research

Government of Canada

Criterion referenced fitness standards - a minimal level score for selected fitness variables that meet acceptable standards for good health.

Table 17.1: Description of different youth fitness tests, simplified

Fitness Component	AAHPER 1958	AAHPER 1975	AAHPER 1988
Cardiorespiratory endurance	600-yd (550-m) walk/run	600-yd (550-m) walk/run	1-mile (1.6-km) run/walk
Body composition	None	None	Skinfolds sum
Flexibility	None	None	Sit-and-reach
Abdominal muscular Strength & endurance	Sit-ups (straight leg)	Sit-ups (bent knee)	Sit-ups (crunches)
Upper body muscular Strength & endurance	Pull-ups	Pull-ups (boys) Flexed armhang (girls)	Pull-ups

---

Table 17.1: Description of different youth fitness tests, cont'd

Fitness Component	AAHPER 1958	AAHPER 1975	AAHPER 1988
Anaerobic power	Standing long jump	Standing long jump	None
Speed	50-yd (45.0-m) dash	50-yd (45.0-m) dash	None
Agility	Shuttle run	Shuttle run	None
Motor Skill	Softball throw	None	None

Body Fat

From 1960's - 1980's there has been an increase in skinfold thickness in children aged 6-11.

Obesity incidence in this population has increased from 17.6% to 27.1% in this time period.

Causes for the increased fat content of children are

- ↓ Physical activity
- ↑ Television viewing

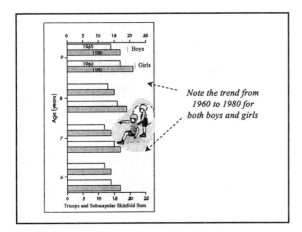

Note the trend from 1960 to 1980 for both boys and girls

Strength

American children have poor muscular strength, especially for the upper body.

Problem: *relationship between musular strength and endurance to scores on the flexed arm hang and pull-up are not well validated*

Based on 1985 testing:

- *40% of boys* aged 6-12 could not complete more than 1 pull-up
- *70% of girls* aged 6-12 could not complete more than 1 pull-up
- *45% of boys* and *55% of girls* aged 6-14 could not hold their chins over ar aised bar for more than 10s

Aerobic Capacity

Performance in the 1mile run field test has declined from 1980 to 1985 by approximately 10%. In addition, American children score worse than children from Europe, Great Britain, Australia and Canada.

Coronary Artery Disease

~ *40%* of children ages 5-8 show at least *1 risk factor* for heart disease
(high cholesterol, physical inactivity, obesity, hypertension)

Coronary artery disease is now recognized as a pediatric disease

---

Some reasons for the concern over the cardiovascular health of our children are:

- ☿ CHD takes over 20 yrs to develop
- ☿ Children are *more fat* and *less fit* than 20 years ago
- ☿ 30-35% of school-aged children are at risk for CHD
- ☿ 50% of children are overweight
- ☿ 42% of children have high blood cholesterol
- ☿ 28% of children have high blood pressure
- ☿ The average 2-5 year-old watches 22 hr of television/week. 6-11 year olds watch 20 hr/week
- ☿ 11 million children in the US are considered obese

Growth and Development

Children do not grow at a uniform rate throughout the course of their development.

The most rapid increase in height and weight occurs during **puberty**, and is referred to as the *pubertal growth spurt*

The most rapid rate of growth occurs during the adolescent years, and is referred to as the *peak height velocity (PHV)*.

Girls tend to be slightly taller and heavier than boys from years 2-10, and PHV occurs 2 years earlier in girls than boys

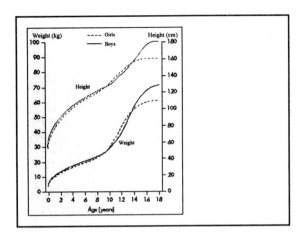

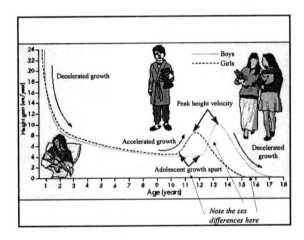

Note the sex
differences here

Assessment of Maturation

As children mature at different rates, chronological age is not a good gauge of physical development or maturation.

Tanner stage of sexual maturation

STAGE	Description
1	Absence of development of any secondary sex characterstics
2	Initial elevation of breast in girls and enlargement of the genitals in boys ; For both sexes, pubic hair begins to grow
3 & 4	Pubic hair becomes coarser and begins to curl Relative enlargement of larynx in boys Increase in pelvic diameter begins in girls
5	Adult maturation; Mature spermatozoa are present in males ; Full reproductivity in women Axially hair is present, and sweat and sebaceous glands are very active in both sexes

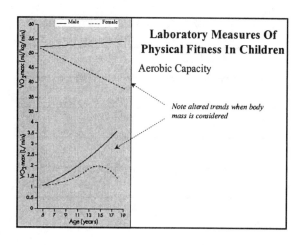

Laboratory Measures Of Physical Fitness In Children

Aerobic Capacity

Note altered trends when body mass is considered

Training Considerations

Even when controlling for maturation, it is clear that children can adapt to endurance training

Physiologic changes in children resulting from training and growth and maturation

Characteristic	Change
Heart rate, resting and submaximal	Decrease
Arterial blood pressure, maximal	Increase
Minute ventilation, maximal	Increase
Oxygen uptake, maximal (L/min)	Increase
Blood and muscle lactate, maximal	Increase
Muscular strength	Increase
Anaerobic power (Watts/kg)	Increase

Anaerobic Capacity

Children have a distinctly lower anaerobic capacity compared to adolescents and adults.

- Low levels of male reproductive hormones
- low glycolytic capacity
- lower lactate production
- decreased buffer capacity
- decreased rates of glycolgenolysis
- lower lactate threshold

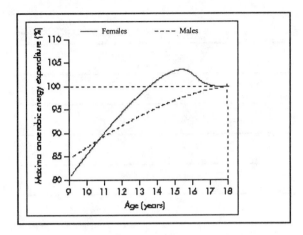

Thermoregulation

Children are not as effective in dissipating heat as adults:

- produce more heat relative to body mass
- lower sweat rates at rest and during exercise
- greater energy expenditure during exercise
- lower cardiac output relative to metabolic intensity
- rely more on convective heat loss than evaporative cooling

Defining Aging

A manifestation of biological events that occur over time.

The **natural lifes pan** is suggested to be the age of 85.

Life expectancy is the average, statistically predicted length of life for an individual.

- 71 years for men of developed countries
- 78 years for women of developed countries

It is estimated that in the near future 50% of all deaths will occur after the age of 80 years

Unfortunately, a large percentage of today's elderly live their last years of life in ill health. Thus, they do not have a *healthy life* that spans as much of their life span as could be possible.

The quality of life is also important. This is best reflected in the ability of an individual to perform activities of daily living (ADL's)

Longevity refers to the duration of life, and is dependent on:
- Heredity
- Environmental factors
- Good medical and health services
- Individual hygene and health habits

Effects of exercise and age on select body systems, simplified

Body System	Exercise	Aging
Circulatory		
VO_2max	Increase	Decrease
HRmax	Increase	Decrease
Cardiac Output, maximal	Increase	Decrease
Vascular resistance	Decrease	Increase
Blood pressure	Same or Decrease	Increase
Blood Components		
Total cholesterol	?	Increase
Triglycerides	Decrease	Increase
LDL cholesterol	?	Increase ?
HDL cholesterol	Increase	Decrease ?

Effects of exercise and age on select body systems, cont'd

Body System	Exercise	Aging
Musckuloskeletal		
Muscular strength	Increase	Decrease
Muscular endurance	Increase	Unchanged
Flexibility	Increase	Decrease
Bone mineral	Increase	Decrease
Lean body mass	Increase	Decrease
Adipose tissue	Decrease	Increase
Regulatory systems		
Basal metabolic rate	Increase	Decrease
Sleep	Increase ?	Decrease
Anxiety/Depression	Decrease?	Increase ?
Cognitive functioning	Increase	Decrease ?

Maximal Oxygen Uptake (VO$_2$max)

Decreased VO$_2$max

Aging associated decreases in maximal cardio-respiratory endurance

↓ Cardiovascular function
↓ Cardiac output
↓ Blood volume   ↓ Stroke volume
  ↓ ejection fraction
  ↓ ventricular filling
  ↓ myocardial compliance and elasticity

↓ Ventilatory and pulmonary function
↑ VE/Q mismatch
↑ Work of breathing
  ↓ Respiratory muscle strength/endurance
  ↓ Lung compliance and elasticity
  ↑ Closing volume

✦ *VO$_2$max decreases 8-10%/decade after age 30*
✦ *VO$_2$max can be equally improved with training in the elderly as it is in youth*

Pulmonary Changes with Age

Structural & functional changes to the pulmonary system with age

Body System	Aging
Structural changes	
Alveolar elastic recoil	Decrease
Respiratory muscle strength	Decrease
Alveolar surface area	Decrease
Pulmonary blood volume	Decrease
Residual lung volume	Increase
Functional changes	
VEmax	Decrease
Expiratory flow rate	Decrease
Maximal voluntary ventilation (MVV)	Decrease
Vital capacity	Decrease

Musculoskeletal System

By age 90, 32% of women and 17% of men will have sustained a hip fracture.

Regular physical activity can decrease the rate of age-related bone mineral loss

Adolescent male
Adolescent female
30 year old - active
30 year old - inactive

-20   -15   -10   -5   0
% Decrease in bone mineral

Muscular Strength

Declines after ~ age 40, with an accelerated decline after age 60.

As with VO_2max, strength training can increase muscular strength similar to that in youth

Arthritis

Osteoarthritis - degenerative joint disease, caused by the wearing away of cartilage.

Rheumatoid arthritis - inflammation of the membrane surrounding joints.

Exercise (eg. swimming) is beneficial to the individual with arthritis because it relieves pain and joint stiffness

Chapter 17

Environmental Physiology

Section I: Exercise When Exposed to Altered Pressure

Exercise at Increased Altitude

As altitude increases, there is a decrease in pressure. This reduced pressure causes air molecules to be more dispersed. Thus, for a given air volume, even though the relative presence (*gas fraction*) of a gas remains the same, there is less of a given gas.

For example,

Sea level
PO_2 in air = 760 mmHg x 0.2093 = 159 mmHg

At Pikes Peak, CO (4,000 m or 14,300 ft)
PO_2 in air = 430 mmHg x 0.2093 = 90 mmHg

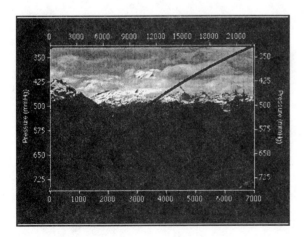

meters	feet	Pressure (Torr)	P_IO_2 (Torr)	P_AO_2 (Torr)	SaO_2 (%)
5250	17500	392	70	50	80
				55	82
4500	15000	431	80	60	84
			90		86
3750	12500	473		65	
			100	70	88
3000	10000	520		75	90
			110		
2250	7500	572		80	92
			120	85	
1500	5000	629			94
			130	90	96
750	2500	691		95	
			140		98
				100	
0	0	760	150		100

1 Torr = 1 mmHg ; 1 m = 3.28 ft ; $P_B = 760 [e^{-(m/7924)}]$; $P_IO_2 = (P_B - 47) \times 0.2093$;
$P_AO_2 \sim (P_B - 47) \times 0.146$; SaO_2 approximated from $\%O_2$-Hb dissociation curve

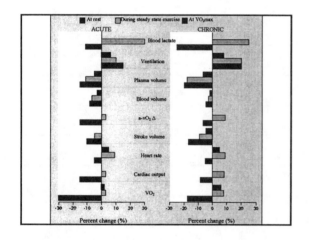

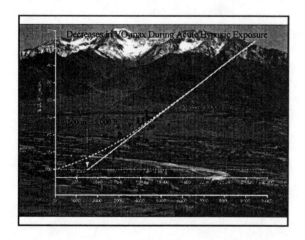

Decreases in VO_2max During Acute Hypoxic Exposure

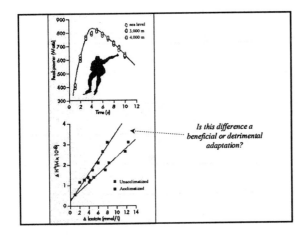

Is this difference a beneficial or detrimental adaptation?

Does living at altitude improve exercise tolerance at altitude? Yes,

- VO$_2$max decrement is not as large
- Ventilation is higher
- Maximal blood lactate is lower
- AMS symptoms are less severe

Does training at altitude improve exercise tolerance at sea level? ???

This question has not adequately been answered. However, there are recent findings that may indicate a benefit of sleeping at altitude (> 7,000 ft) and training at low-moderate altitude (< 7,000 ft).

Exercise During Hyperbaria

Hyperbaria refers to exposure to increased pressure above 1 atmosphere (atm = 760 mmHg).

For example;
When submerged in sea water, pressure increases by 1 atm every 10 m. In fresh water, the pressure change is not as great and approximates 10.4 m.

Physiological changes associated with hyperbaria include,

- ↓ cutaneous blood flow
- ↑ central blood volume and venous return
- ↓ heart rate
- ↑ diuresis
- ↑ VO$_2$

3

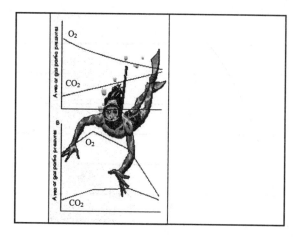

Section II: Exercise And Thermal Stress

Dehydration - decrease in total body water. Occurs at a faster rate during exercise in hot and/or humid environments

for example,

sweat rates can to 2-3 L/Hr

Deleterious effects of dehydration on exercise occur with as little as fluid loss equal to 2% body weight.

For a 70 kg male; 70 x 0.02 = 1.4 kg ~ 1.4 L

This could occur with as little as 30 min of exercise!!!!

Hyperthermia - increased body temperature resulting from body heat storage

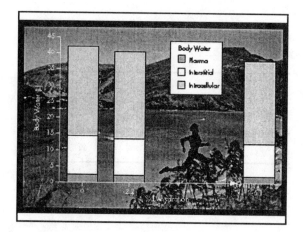

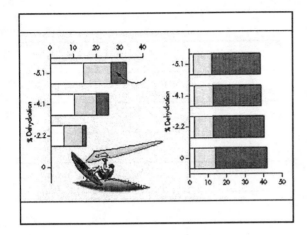

Physiological changes during dehydration

- ✴ ↑ Core temperature
- ✴ ↓ Plasma volume
- ✴ ↓ Venous return
- ✴ ↓ Stroke volume
- ✴ ↑ Heart rate
- ✴ ↓ Cardiac output
- ✴ ↑ a-vO$_2$Δ
- ✴ ↓ Skin blood flow

- ✴ ↑ Catecholamines
- ✴ ↑ Blood lactate
- ✴ ↑ VO$_2$
- ✴ CNS dysfunction
- ✴ ↓ Exercise tolerance
- ✴ ↓ Sweat rate
- ✴ ↓ Evaporative cooling

Improving Exercise Tolerance During Heat Exposure

≋ Fluid intake (pre-during and post-exercise)

≋ Do not rely on thirst mechanism

≋ Complete heat acclimation or acclimatization

Acclimation - chronic adaptations induced by exposure to artificial environmental conditions
(eg. environmental chambers, sauna, exercise)

Acclimatization - chronic adaptations induced by exposure to foreign a foreign climat
(eg. geographical relocation)

Chronic adaptations to exercise and exercise in a hot environment that improve acclimation to exercise in the heat

Acclimation/Adaptation	Physiological Benefit
Plasma Volume	↑ Blood Volume
	↑ Venous return
	↑ Cardiac output
	↓ Submaximal heart rate
	Sustained sweat response
	↑ Capacity for evaporative cooling
Earlier onset of sweating	Improved evaporative cooling
Osmolality of sweat	Electrolyte conservation (mainly Na⁺)
Muscle glycogenolysis	↓ Likelihood for muscle fatigue

Heat Illness, Heat Exhaustion and Heat Stroke

These conditions are more severe clinical manifestations of heat exposure.

Heat Exhaustion - the decreased cardiovascular function that accompanies dehydration and mild hyperthermia

Heat Stroke - when heat stress continues, or is worsened beyond that of heat exhaustion (core temp > 39.5 °C), physiological symptoms progress to CNS dysfunction - *disorientation, confusion, psychoses*

Heat exhaustion and heat stroke are both **heat illnesses**. However, heat stroke can be potentially lethal due potential organ damage and failure.

Evaluating Environmental Conditions For Risk of Heat Injury

An index has been developed that incorporates all contributors to thermal heat stress - **Wet Bulb Globe Index** (WBGI)

Dry bulb temperature - measure of air temperature

Black bulb temperature - measure of the potential for radiative heat gain

Wet bulb temperature - measure of the potential for evaporative cooling

$$WBGI = (0.7 \times Tw) + (0.2 \times Tb) + (0.1 \times Td)$$

The relative risks for heat injury at different ranges of the WBGI	
WGBI	**Physiological Benefit**
23-28	**High risk for heat injury: red flag** Make runners aware that heat injury is possible, especially for those with a history of susceptibility to heat illness
18-23	**Moderate risk for heat injury:** amber flag Make runners aware that the risk for heat injury will increase during the race
< 18	**Low risk for heat injury: green flag** Make runners aware that although the risk is low, there is still a possibility for heat injury to occur
< 10	**Possible risk for hypothermia: white flag** Make runners aware that conditions may cause excessive heat loss from the body, especially for individuals who will have slow race times and when conditions are wet and windy

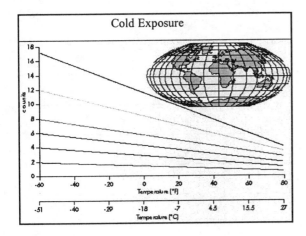

Cold Exposure

Section III: Human Function and Performance During Gravitational Challenge

Microgravity

The early space programs of the USA and Russia revealed that prolonged exposure to microgravity was detrimental to human physiology.

The earth has a reference gravitational force = 1 g

The moon's gravitational force = 0.17g

Outside a planetary orbit (eg. Space Shuttle), gravitatonal force = 0g

Research models that have been used to mimic physiological responses to microgravity are,

head-down bed rest   lower body negative pressure   tilt testing

Physiological Effects of Exposure to Microgravity

- 🜨 Muscle atrophy
- 🜨↓ Bone mineral
- 🜨 ↓ Muscle enzymes
- 🜨 ↓ Blood volume
- 🜨 ↑ Diuresis
- 🜨 ↑ Heart rate
- 🜨 ↓ Stroke volume
- 🜨 Compromised regulation of peripheral blood vessels and vascular resistance

---

Section IV: Exercise And Air Pollution

Pollutant	Upper Healthy Limit	Detriment
Carbn monoxide (CO)	9 ppm	Greater affinity for Hb than O2
Carbon dioxide (CO₂)	----	Hyperventilation, acid-base, headache
Ozone (O₃)	0.12 ppm	Decreased lung function, headache
Sulphuric acid (H₂CO₄)	----	Irritates upper respiratory tract
Sulfur oxide (SO₂)	0.14 ppm	Exercicse-induced bronchospasm
Nitrogen dioxide (NO₂)	----	Lung irritant
Suspended particles	150 μg/m³	Aggravation of asthma and obstructuve lung disease

Chapter 18

Gender and Exercise

A General Comparison of Male and Female Structure and Function

This is difficult to do, as many men and women differ to representative averages. However, there are differences between genders in features such as:

- Body composition
- Hematology
- Maximal cardiorespiratory capacity(VO_2max)
- Pulmonary function
- Endocrinology
- Substrate use during exercise

VARIABLE	Female Age 20-30 yrs	Male Age 20-30 yrs
%Fat	27%	15%
LBM	49 kg	61 kg
[Hb]	120 – 140 g/L	140 – 160 g/L
Hct	40 – 44%	42 – 46%
Blood volume	4.5 – 5.0 L	5.0 – 6.0 L
VO2max	3.0 – 3.5 L/min	3.5 – 4.0 L/min
VC	4 – 5 L	5 – 6 L
RV	1.2 – 1.6 L	1.6 – 2.0 L
[Estradiol]	30 – 200 pg/mL	< 5 pg/mL
[Progesterone]	0.15 – 15 ng/mL	< 0.5 ng/mL
[Testoserone]	< 500 pg/mL	500 10,000 pg/mL

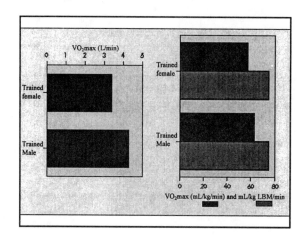

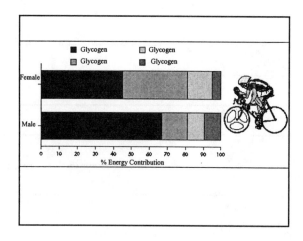

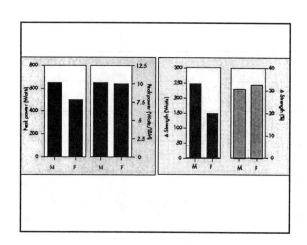

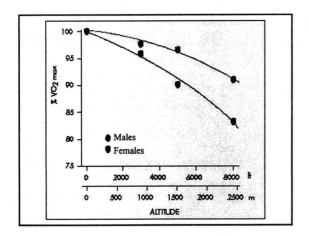

_____

_____

_____

_____

_____

_____

_____

Chapter 19

Exercise, Health and Disease Prevention

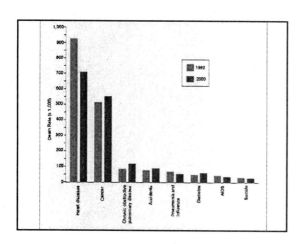

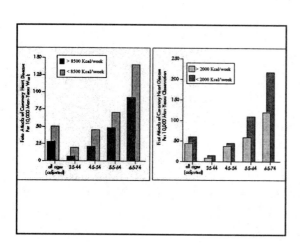

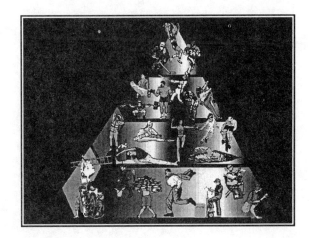

_____

_____

_____

_____

_____

_____

_____

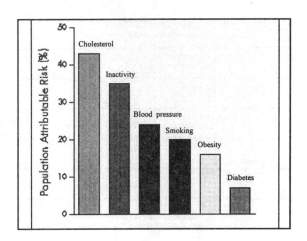

_____

_____

_____

_____

_____

_____

_____

Chapter 20

Clinical Exercise Physiology

Uses of Clinical Exercise Testing

- Diagnose the presence and severity of disease

- Establish the functional capacity of an individual

- Evaluate medical therapy

Exercise testing is used in a variety of clinical settings that are summarized in Table 16.1.

The importance of exercise in the *prevention, diagnosis, and rehabilitation* of the most common and deadly diseases of today's society can not be overemphasized.

Use of clinical exercise testing, simplified

Exercise Testing in Clinical Practice
Apparently Healthy
Determine functional capacity
Screen for disease
Develop exercise prescription
High-Risk Individuals
Diagnostic tool
After myocardial infarction
Evaluate medical therapy
Known Disease
Determine functional capacity
After myocardial infarction or heart surgery
Diabetes

Contraindications of Clinical Exercise Testing

Due to the potential for exercise to pose a too greater risk to life or injury in individuals with disease or specific symptoms of disease or ill health, guidelines exist for when to not conduct an exercise test.

Some of the contraindications to exercise testing include:

- Recent MI
- Unstable angina
- Third-degree AVblock
- Acute congestive heart failure
- Severe aortic stenosis
- Aneurysm
- Acite infection
- Significant emotional distress

Knowledge of electrocardiography (ECG) is essential in clinical exercise physiology.

The 12-lead ECG is a vital component of the evaluation of heart function during the exercise test.

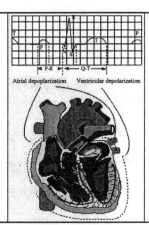

Interpretation of the 12-Lead Electrocardiogram

You should use a consistent approach every time you evaluate any ECG.

Rate   **Rhythm**   **Axis**

Tachycardia - HR > 100 b/min

Bradycardia - HR < 60 b/min

Arrhythmias - abnormal or inconsistent cardiac rhythms

Axis - refers to the direction of depolarization of the mean QRS vector (0 - +90°)

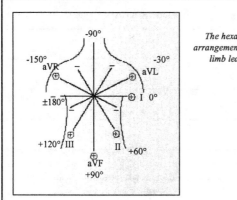

The hexaxial arrangement of the limb leads

Quadrant identification for determination of axis

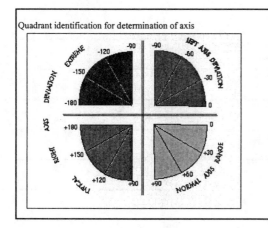

ST-Segment Depression

The hallmark of myocardial ischemia. Caused by the reduction in arterial blood supply to region(s) of the myocardium, which in turn alters the myocardial membrane potential, causing the ST segment depression.

Downsloping   ***Horizontal***   ***Upsloping***

Myocardial Infarction - myocardial cell death resulting from excess ischemia.

The ability to detect myocardial ischemia on the ECG is increased by the inclusion of the precordial leads.

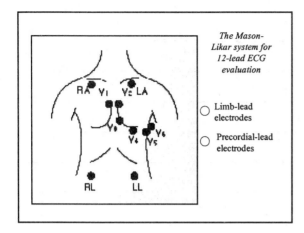

The Mason-Likar system for 12-lead ECG evaluation

○ Limb-lead electrodes

○ Precordial-lead electrodes

Some Common Clinical Exercise Test Protocols

Bruce   ***Naughton-Balke***   ***Balke***

The Bruce protocol

Stage	Duration (min)	Speed (m/Hr)	Grade (%)	METs
1	3:00	1.7	10.0	4.6
2	3:00	2.5	12.0	7.0
3	3:00	3.4	14.0	10.1
4	3:00	4.2	16.0	12.9
5	3:00	5.0	18.0	15.0
6	3:00	5.5	20.0	16.9
7	3:00	6.0	22.0	19.1

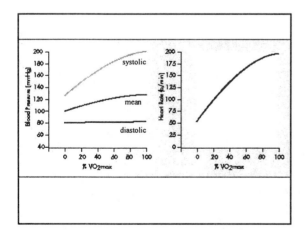

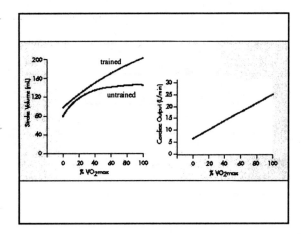

Predictive Value of Clinical Exercise Testing

How accurately an exercise test correctly identifies an individual with coronary artery disease. The predictive value is estimated using **Baye's Theorum** in the calculation of test *sensitivity* and *specificity*.

Sensitivity - % of individuals who are tested that will have an abnormal test (~71%). Thus, there is a 29% likelihood for a *false negative* test.

Specificity - % of individuals who are tested that will have a normal test (~73%). Thus, there is a 27% likelihood for a *false positive* test.

Note: a positive test is one that detects disease when it is present